Cannabis Grow Guide Book

Grow Top-Shelf Weed at Home—Step-by-Step Blueprint for Big Yields, Potent Buds, and Indoor/ Outdoor Success

by

Jake Lawson

Cannabis Grow Guide Book : Grow Top-Shelf Weed at Home—Step-by-Step Blueprint for Big Yields, Potent Buds, and Indoor/Outdoor Success

Table of Contents

INTRODUCTION

Growing cannabis at home has shifted from being a niche hobby to a widely embraced passion for many. Whether you're curious about starting your first grow or have some experience under your belt, this guide is designed to provide you with a clear path toward cultivating high-quality marijuana in your own space. The journey of cannabis cultivation involves both art and science, blending knowledge with hands-on practice, and that's exactly what you'll find throughout this book.

It's important to recognize that growing cannabis isn't just about planting seeds and letting nature take its course. There's a real depth of technique and understanding behind producing buds that are not just potent but also flavorful and visually appealing. Many growers have found that satisfying and rewarding cultivation comes from mastering some key principles—those that are easier to grasp than you might expect. By delivering straightforward advice and practical steps, this book aims to strip away the confusion often associated with cannabis growing.

One of the biggest hurdles beginners face is where to start. The abundance of information out there can quickly feel overwhelming, especially when you run into conflicting advice. This book functions as a comprehensive blueprint, guiding you step by step without unnecessary jargon or vague generalities. We focus on providing solid, hands-on guidance that allows you to make confident decisions from seed selection all the way through harvest and beyond.

Safety and legality are foundational elements of responsible cannabis cultivation. Growing marijuana at home isn't just about the science of the plant; it's equally about respecting laws and ensuring your personal setup adheres to local regulations. Understanding these boundaries upfront will help you avoid potential problems while fostering a positive growing environment. The approach here emphasizes not only successful cultivation but also legal and ethical practices that contribute to the responsible normalization of cannabis growing.

The ideal grower is someone who's curious, willing to invest time and attention, and eager to learn from each stage of the process. Whether you're aiming for a small personal stash or a more substantial harvest, this book's guidance adjusts to fit your goals. High-quality cannabis production doesn't just rely on luck; it relies on knowledge, observation, and a bit of patience. You'll find encouragement to develop these traits through clear explanations, motivation to keep going during tougher moments, and descriptions that help you visualize what your plants should look and feel like at every phase.

It's also worth noting that cannabis cultivation combines both indoor and outdoor opportunities, each with unique challenges and rewards. While this introduction won't dive deep into those specifics, it sets the stage for you to explore different growing styles later in the book. You'll discover how factors like environment, light, and space influence your choices and ultimate success. Understanding the bigger picture will help you pick a growing path that matches your lifestyle and resources.

Throughout this book, the language will maintain a balance between instructional and motivational. You won't just get dry facts; you'll find explanations that inspire confidence to try new techniques and adapt as you learn. Growing cannabis at home is a personal journey, and the right mindset can make all the difference. With the encouragement to observe, experiment, and refine your approach, this book sets you up for not just one successful crop, but for ongoing improvement over time.

Starting your grow means understanding the cannabis plant itself—the various strains, chemical compounds like THC and CBD, as well as the anatomy and growth cycle. While those topics are discussed in detail in upcoming chapters, this introduction gives you a sense of why these basics matter for any grower. The plant's biology directly impacts decisions like lighting, nutrients, and harvesting. Grasping this connection early on makes the technical steps feel more intuitive and manageable.

One of the most exciting parts of cultivation is watching your plants thrive and respond to care. From the initial sprouting of seedlings to the final flame of trichomes ready for harvest, cannabis cultivation encourages patience and attentiveness. Each plant is unique, reacting to conditions in its own way, which is part of the fascination. By learning key markers of healthy growth and potential problems, you'll develop an almost instinctual ability to nurture rewarding crops.

This book recognizes that not every grower has lavish setups or commercial ambitions. Many home cultivators value simplicity and cost-effectiveness without sacrificing quality. As you proceed, you'll see how thoughtful choices in equipment and methods make a big difference, regardless of budget. Starting small with the right fundamentals can lead to impressive results over time. And if you decide to upgrade your grow space or techniques down the road, you'll understand how to make those improvements strategically.

Another vital aspect of home growing is the post-harvest process, which includes drying, curing, and storing your cannabis. These steps have a significant impact on flavor, potency, and overall quality. Many new growers underestimate how much attention these phases deserve. This book lays the groundwork by emphasizing that quality cultivation extends beyond the flowering stage—a high-quality grower treats the entire lifecycle of the plant with care.

As you embark on the cannabis growing journey, remember that challenges and setbacks are part of the experience. Problems like pests, nutrient imbalances, and environmental fluctuations are common even among seasoned cultivators. What sets successful growers apart is how they recognize and address these issues promptly while maintaining a proactive mindset. The knowledge you acquire here will equip you to troubleshoot effectively and keep your plants thriving.

Bringing everything together, this book offers an accessible, thorough exploration of cannabis cultivation aimed at helping you build confidence from the ground up. You don't have to be a horticultural expert to produce quality flowers. With the right guidance, patience, and persistence, you'll transform your enthusiasm into a rewarding, productive home grow. Welcome to a journey where science meets craft, and where the satisfaction of cultivating your own cannabis becomes a reality.

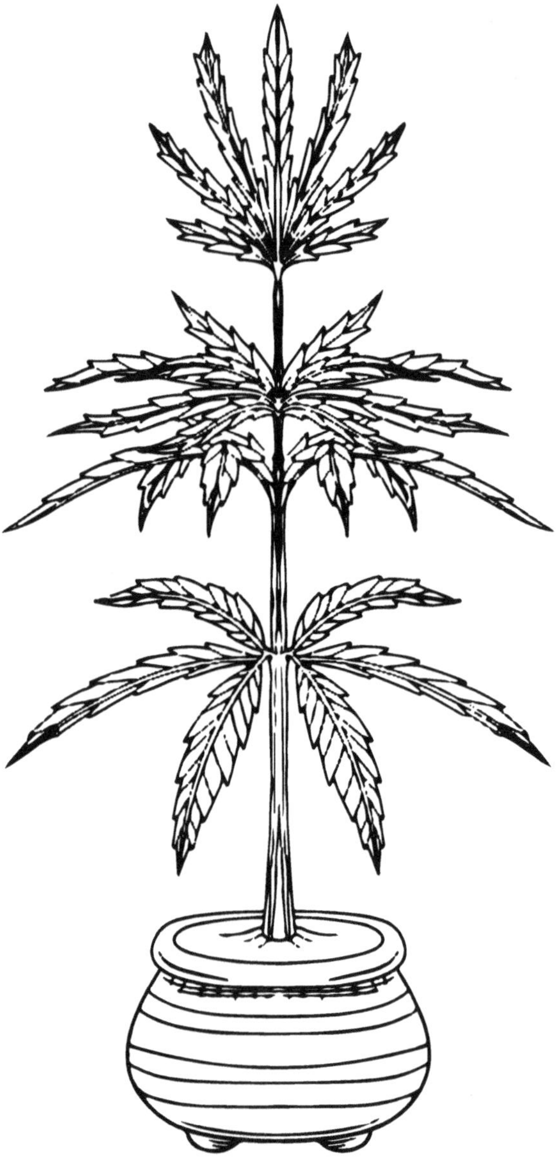

Chapter 1
Cannabis 101

Getting started with cannabis growing means first understanding what sets this plant apart: its varieties, components, and biological makeup. Cannabis comes mainly in three types—indica, sativa, and hybrid—and each brings distinct growth patterns, effects, and cultivation needs that influence what you can expect from your crop. Key compounds like THC and CBD also play a huge role, not just in the plant's effects but in how you handle its growth and harvesting. Plus, knowing the anatomy of cannabis—from roots and stems to leaves and flowers—gives you an edge when it's time to nurture healthy plants. This chapter lays the groundwork by highlighting these essentials, preparing you to grow with confidence before diving into the detailed steps ahead.

Understanding Cannabis Types: Indica, Sativa, Hybrid

When starting your journey into cannabis cultivation, understanding the basic types of cannabis plants is crucial. The three primary categories you'll hear about are Indica, Sativa, and Hybrid. Each category has unique characteristics that affect everything from plant growth to the effects of the final product. Knowing how these types differ can guide you in selecting the right strain for your growing environment and desired outcome.

Indica strains tend to originate from regions with cooler climates and higher altitudes, such as the Hindu Kush mountains near Afghanistan. They're often shorter, bushier plants with broader leaves. Compared to their Sativa counterparts, Indicas typically grow quicker and finish flowering in less time, making them attractive options for growers who want a faster turnaround. Their denser and more compact bud structure is another hallmark, which can translate to higher yields per plant under the right conditions.

But beyond just physical characteristics, Indicas are popularly associated with relaxing, sedative effects. Many consumers use Indica strains for stress relief, pain management, or to support sleep. This is partly due to their cannabinoid and terpene profiles, which often create a heavier, calming sensation. As a grower, this influences the types of strains you might focus on depending on your end-user needs. Whether you're cultivating for medicinal users or personal relaxation, understanding these traits will affect your choice.

Sativa strains arise from tropical or equatorial climates, such as parts of Central America and Southeast Asia. Physically, Sativas are taller and lankier with narrow leaves, often reaching impressive heights outdoors. They typically have longer flowering times, which means they require more patience and sometimes specialized environmental control indoors. Their buds tend to be less dense and more elongated compared to Indicas.

The effects of Sativa strains are often described as uplifting, energetic, and cerebral. This makes them popular for daytime use or for creative pursuits. They may boost focus and enhance mood without the heavy sedation you might experience with Indicas. As a cultivator, the longer growth and flowering period can require careful planning, especially if you're working within space or time constraints. Managing height and light exposure becomes essential with these fast-growing, towering plants.

Hybrid strains are exactly what their name suggests: a blend of Indica and Sativa genetics. These plants are bred to combine desirable traits from both types, leading to a broad spectrum of characteristics depending on the specific parent strains involved. Hybrids can lean more Indica or more Sativa, or sit neatly in the middle, providing a balance of effects and growth patterns suited to different preferences.

Because hybrids offer the best of both worlds, they have become some of the most popular strains on the market today. Many cultivators appreciate the flexibility hybrids provide in tailoring the plant's effects, yield, and flowering times to their particular needs. The genetic diversity found in hybrids also opens up exciting possibilities for selective breeding and fine-tuning strain characteristics, allowing growers to experiment with new flavors, potencies, and plant structures.

Physically, hybrids often inherit medium stature and leaf shape, but this can vary widely. Depending on the genetic dominance, you could end up with a bushy, quick-flowering plant or something taller with a longer bloom time. This variability means it's essential to research individual hybrid strains carefully, especially when thinking about your grow setup, available space, and the timeline you have in mind.

One important note for growers: while Indica, Sativa, and Hybrid labels help categorize cannabis, modern breeding has blurred the lines significantly. Many strains have been bred extensively over decades, with genetics crossing back and forth. What's branded as Indica or Sativa might actually carry a mixture of traits from both sides. This makes it vital to look at the specific genetics and not rely solely on the category label when planning your grow.

The chemical profile of these categories also varies. While THC and CBD levels depend mostly on individual strains rather than just type, some trends exist. Indica strains might have a slightly higher CBD content on average, contributing to their more calming effects, while Sativas frequently feature higher THC levels, creating their characteristic energizing qualities. Hybrids can fall anywhere on this spectrum, depending on the blend.

Terpenes—the aromatic oils found in cannabis—play a huge role in how these plants smell, taste, and affect the user. Indicas often have earthier, muskier scents with notes of pine or spice. Sativas tend toward citrus, fruity, or floral aromas that feel lighter and more vibrant. Hybrids can combine these terpene profiles in countless ways, offering unique sensory experiences that can influence growth decisions, such as strain selection based on desired aromas or flavor for personal use or marketability.

For beginners, a hybrid strain can be an ideal starting point because it offers a mix of manageable growth traits and versatile effects. You often get a balance of plant size, flowering time, and a breadth of effects that are neither too heavy nor too stimulating. This middle ground can reduce some of the pressures you might feel when choosing strictly Indica or Sativa, both of which might demand more specific environmental controls or patience.

Experienced growers, however, may prefer to dive deeper into the distinctions and tailor their cultivation techniques to match the particular needs of Indica or Sativa strains. For example, Indicas respond well to pruning and training methods that maximize compact growth and light exposure. Sativas, on the other hand, often need more space and support to handle their height and longer flowering time. Knowing these nuances can make a big difference in optimizing yield and plant health.

Ultimately, understanding these types isn't just about classification—it shapes the entire cultivation journey. From choosing seeds and planning your grow area to managing light cycles and nutrients, the core type of your cannabis plant influences every decision you make. This knowledge arms you with confidence and precision throughout the growing process, increasing your chances of a successful, rewarding harvest.

As you move forward in this guide, keep in mind that the cannabis landscape is continually evolving. New hybrids emerge, breeding techniques improve, and growers worldwide experiment with fresh genetics. Staying informed about strain types and how they perform in various environments keeps your grow game strong. Whether you dream of a soothing Indica for evening relaxation or an uplifting Sativa for social moments, your understanding of these foundational categories sets the stage for excellent cultivation results.

THC vs. CBD: What Matters for Cannabis Growers

When diving into the world of cannabis cultivation, understanding the difference between THC and CBD is crucial. These two cannabinoids are the stars of the show, each carrying distinct effects and implications that every grower should consider. While many focus heavily on THC due to its psychoactive properties, CBD is gaining equal footing because of its medicinal potential and popularity among consumers seeking non-intoxicating benefits. For growers, knowing which cannabinoid to emphasize can shape the entire growing process, from selecting seeds to optimizing conditions for the best yield.

THC, or tetrahydrocannabinol, is the primary psychoactive compound in cannabis. It's responsible for that characteristic "high," affecting mood, perception, and cognition. Most recreational users target strains with high THC levels to get that powerful euphoric sensation. But from a grower's perspective, cultivating high-THC plants often demands not only a good grasp of genetics but also meticulous care during each growth phase. THC concentrations can fluctuate significantly based on environmental factors, nutrient balance, and harvest timing. Therefore, if the goal is to maximize THC content, growers need to focus heavily on these variables.

On the other hand, CBD, or cannabidiol, doesn't produce a high but offers many therapeutic benefits like pain relief, anti-anxiety effects, and anti-inflammatory properties. This has made it incredibly popular for medicinal use and has opened up a growing market for CBD-rich cannabis products. For growers, producing CBD-dominant plants involves different strategies compared to THC-heavy crops. Selective breeding plays a major role here; CBD-rich strains often come from genetics that either suppress THC or balance both cannabinoids to achieve the desired effect.

One of the biggest considerations for growers is market demand. Recreational consumers may prefer high-THC strains, but medical users and wellness-oriented consumers often seek out high-CBD cultivars. This demand can influence what seeds you decide to grow. It's important to align your cultivation goals with what your intended consumers are looking for, whether it's a potent psychoactive experience or therapeutic relief without intoxication.

Beyond market trends, the cultivation process itself varies between THC and CBD dominant plants. Although both cannabinoids develop within the plant's resinous trichomes, the pathways for their biosynthesis are genetically controlled. This means that environmental stressors like temperature, humidity, and light can impact THC and CBD levels differently. For example, some growers report that higher temperatures may degrade THC more readily, while CBD maintains stability under similar conditions. So managing your grow environment isn't just about plant health; it can directly affect the cannabinoid profile of your harvest.

Choosing the right strain or seed is the first step when deciding whether to focus on THC, CBD, or a balanced combination. Many breeders offer specialized seeds tailored for specific cannabinoid ratios. Some strains lean heavily towards THC, others toward CBD, and many hybrids aim for a harmonious mix of both. As you gain experience, exploring these genetic options helps you hone in on a product that suits your preferences and growing conditions. Experimentation is part of the fun here, but starting with well-established genetics can lessen the learning curve.

Another factor to consider is the plant's flowering cycle. While THC and CBD levels both peak during flowering, the timing of harvest can significantly influence the cannabinoid content. Harvesting too early or too late may reduce the potency of either compound. Generally, trichome inspections—checking their color and development—serve as a guide for when cannabinoids are at their peak. Many growers swear by carefully timing harvest based on trichome maturity to balance the ratio of THC to CBD tailored to their desired effects.

For growers concerned about legal restrictions, cannabinoid content carries additional weight. In many places, hemp is defined by law as cannabis containing less than 0.3% THC by dry weight. This makes CBD cultivation within those limits legal in many regions, even where recreational THC-rich cannabis remains restricted. Understanding these thresholds is essential for growers looking to sell their products within regulation. If your plants surpass legal THC limits, this could complicate sales or require separate licensing, so always keep local laws in mind when planning your grow.

Beyond legality, managing cannabinoid content also affects cultivation practices, particularly when it comes to pest control and nutrient management. Some growers have noticed that stress, whether from pests or inconsistent feeding, can alter cannabinoid synthesis. Mild stress might even be used intentionally by experienced cultivators to enhance resin production, but too much stress usually harms cannabinoid potency and flower quality. Maintaining a stable, healthy environment encourages plants to express their genetics optimally.

One increasingly popular technique for influencing the THC vs. CBD balance is the use of specific training and pruning methods. Light stress training and topping can improve airflow and light penetration, potentially boosting resin production and cannabinoid synthesis. However, how these techniques affect THC and CBD ratios specifically isn't fully understood yet. Many growers find that optimizing plant structure supports higher overall potency without sacrificing cannabinoid quality, regardless of whether THC or CBD is the target.

It's also worth noting that THC and CBD work together in what's called the entourage effect, where various cannabinoids and terpenes combine to modify the overall experience. For growers, producing a diverse cannabinoid profile rather than focusing on a single compound might be more beneficial. This could mean cultivating strains that offer a good balance of THC, CBD, and other minor cannabinoids like CBG or CBN. Such complexity in your crop can make your harvest appealing to a wider range of consumers who seek nuanced effects beyond just a THC high or pure CBD relief.

When it comes to processing and finishing your product, THC and CBD content can influence curing techniques too. THC-heavy buds often require careful cure management to preserve potency and aroma, as some cannabinoids are sensitive to light and oxygen. CBD-rich flowers also benefit from a steady curing process but might be more stable during drying. Paying attention to how you store and cure your buds can protect the cannabinoid profile you worked so hard to develop during cultivation.

In essence, the choice between growing for THC, CBD, or a balance of both comes down to your goals, resources, and the audience you aim to serve. Each cannabinoid offers unique challenges and rewards, and understanding their biology and market relevance sets the foundation for successful growing. Whether you want potent psychoactive buds or wellness-focused flowers, aligning your grow practices with the cannabinoid profile is key to producing quality cannabis that meets expectations.

As you move forward in your cultivation journey, keep these points in mind and don't be afraid to experiment within the framework of sound science and legal compliance. Knowledge of THC and CBD isn't just academic—it directly impacts your crop's success and your satisfaction as a grower. Mastering this balance brings you one step closer to perfecting your home-grown cannabis, one plant at a time.

Anatomy of the Cannabis Plant Explained

To truly master cannabis cultivation, getting familiar with the plant's anatomy is a crucial first step. Understanding each part helps you recognize how the plant grows, what it needs to thrive, and where the precious cannabinoids form. Whether you're a beginner or someone with some growing under your belt, grasping the key structures can take your cultivation game up a notch. Let's break down the main components of the cannabis plant—roots, stems, leaves, flowers, and trichomes—and what role each one plays.

Starting beneath the surface, the **root system** anchors your cannabis plant and is responsible for absorbing water and nutrients from the soil or growing medium. Healthy roots are vital because they support overall plant growth and help resist diseases. Roots spread out radially and dip downward in search of moisture and nourishment. A robust root system translates directly into more vigorous plants and ultimately better yields. If your roots struggle with compacted soil, poor drainage, or root rot, the whole plant's performance suffers, no matter how much care you give above.

Moving upward, the **stem** acts as the plant's backbone. It supports leaves, branches, and flowers while serving as the highway for water, nutrients, and sugars traveling between roots and other tissues. The stem's thickness and firmness indicate plant health; a weak stem usually means the plant isn't getting enough light or support. Strong stems help the plant handle bigger buds without snapping under their weight. Plus, the stem plays a role in photosynthesis, particularly with green, healthy outer layers conducting light absorption.

Leaf structure is one of the most recognizable features of cannabis. Cannabis leaves are categorized as *fan leaves* and *sugar leaves*. Fan leaves are large, broad, and arranged symmetrically, often with serrated edges. Their primary job is photosynthesis—converting light into the energy the plant needs to grow. Fan leaves can also help identify the plant's genetic background; for instance, sativa strains typically have longer, thinner leaves, while indicas sport wider, broader ones. Sugar leaves are smaller and grow close to the flowering sites. These are often coated in the sticky resin full of cannabinoids and terpenes that produce the plant's signature scent and effect profile.

The heart of the cannabis plant is the **flowers** or *buds*. These flowering sites hold the highest concentration of cannabinoids, like THC and CBD, making them the most valuable part for both recreational and medicinal users. Buds form on female plants when they enter the flowering phase, triggered by changes in light exposure. They develop from tiny white hairs called pistils, which catch pollen for reproduction but also serve as a handy indicator for growers tracking maturity. As buds mature, they swell and become resinous. Proper care during flowering ensures denser, more potent flowers.

To give a bit more depth, pistils and calyxes make up much of the flower's visible anatomy. Pistils start as bright white hairs that eventually darken, signaling the plant's progress toward harvest readiness. Layers of calyxes, which are small tear-shaped nodules, protect the plant's reproductive organs and produce many of the glandular trichomes where cannabinoids reside.

Speaking of **trichomes**, these tiny, mushroom-shaped glands are arguably the cannabis plant's crown jewels. Found densely covering flowers and even sugar leaves, trichomes manufacture and store cannabinoids and terpenes—the compounds behind the plant's potency, flavor, and aroma. For growers, the appearance and color of trichomes are key harvest indicators. Clear trichomes show the plant isn't quite ready, cloudy ones suggest peak potency, and amber indicates the cannabinoids are beginning to degrade but can yield more relaxing effects. A good understanding of trichome development is essential to harvesting at the ideal time for your desired cannabinoid profile.

Beyond these primary components, cannabis plants produce different **types of leaves and branches** that serve specific purposes. For example, the plant grows numerous secondary branches to increase its bud sites. The way these branches grow and spread is influenced by genetics and pruning techniques you'll explore in other sections. Leaves regulate transpiration, which controls moisture release, and the plant's natural defenses against heat and pests.

It's also important to understand the differences between male and female plants within the anatomy context. Female plants develop the resinous buds everyone covets, whereas male plants produce pollen sacs needed for breeding but rarely for harvest unless seed production is your goal. Male plants typically have fewer leaves and less resin production, so identifying and removing males early helps preserve cannabinoid-rich flowers on female plants.

The anatomy of cannabis doesn't just stop at the visible organs; internal processes such as nutrient transport, photosynthesis, and hormonal regulation work behind the scenes to support growth. However, a grower's visible guide to these processes lies in observing healthy stems, lush fan leaves, robust roots, and well-formed buds.

When you're setting out to cultivate cannabis, learning to recognize the anatomy allows you to diagnose problems quickly and optimize growing conditions. For example, drooping fan leaves might suggest over- or underwatering, and sparse buds could mean insufficient light or nutrient deficiencies. Each component of the plant offers clues you can act on to improve yield and quality.

Throughout the lifecycle, the cannabis plant changes dramatically as it moves from seedling to vegetative growth, then into flowering and finally harvest. Each stage demands specific attention to the plant's anatomical needs. For instance, early on, root and stem development are priorities since they lay the foundation for vigorous growth. Later, the focus shifts toward maximizing bud development, trichome production, and resin quality during flowering.

Getting hands-on experience with cannabis anatomy also builds confidence and intuition for cultivating. As you care for your plants, you'll start predicting what they need just by examining their growth patterns, leaf condition, and flower formation. This practical knowledge is invaluable, especially when it comes to adjusting your environment or nutrient regimen.

In summary, the cannabis plant comprises several critical parts that work together in delicate harmony. From the roots beneath the surface to the trichome-covered buds at the top, each element plays a key role in producing high-quality marijuana. Recognizing these parts and their functions sets a strong foundation for successful growing, helping you nurture your plants with precision and care. As you proceed through this guide, keep the plant's anatomy in mind—you'll be referring back to these concepts time and again while learning how to cultivate cannabis like a pro.

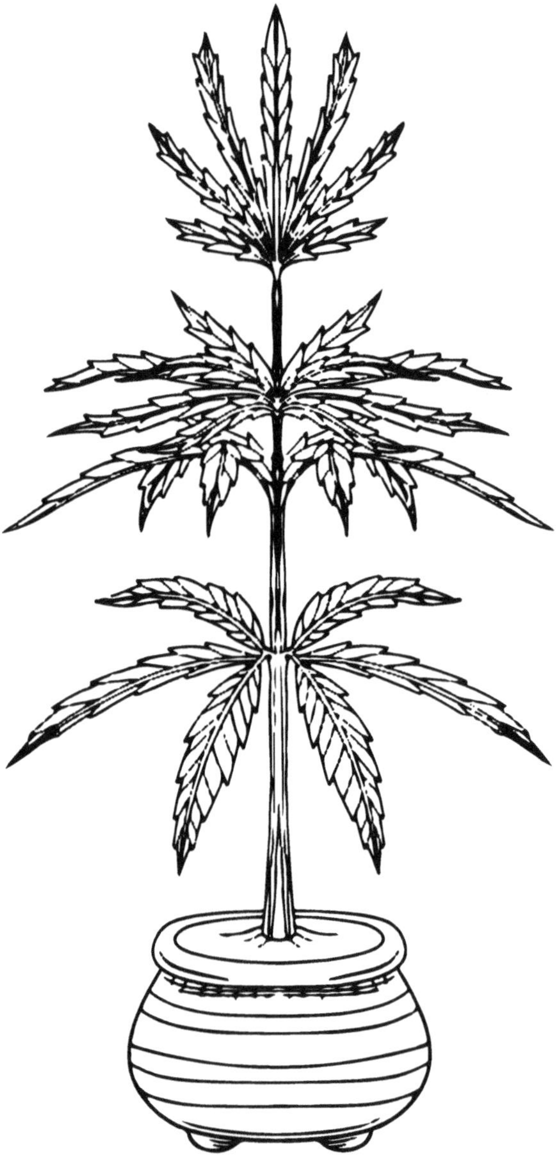

Chapter 2
Choosing Your Grow Style

Deciding on a grow style is a crucial early step that sets the tone for your entire cannabis cultivation journey, and whether you lean toward indoor or outdoor methods depends on your available space, climate, budget, and privacy needs. Indoor growing gives you control over light, temperature, and pests, letting you create an optimal environment year-round, but it often requires a bigger upfront investment and more technical know-how. Outdoor cultivation, on the other hand, lets plants soak up natural sunlight and breathe fresh air, which can lead to bigger yields and vibrant flavors, though it relies heavily on weather and seasonal cycles. Ultimately, picking the right grow style means balancing these pros and cons with your personal goals and circumstances so you can enjoy growing cannabis successfully and sustainably, no matter your experience level.

Indoor vs. Outdoor Growing Overview

When it comes to choosing your grow style, one of the very first big decisions you'll face is whether to cultivate cannabis indoors or outdoors. Each method offers its own unique experience, set of challenges, and opportunities. Understanding the fundamental differences can help you align your growing approach with your goals, space, budget, and climate. Both indoor and outdoor grows have delivered stellar results for countless cultivators, but they do it in very distinct ways.

Indoor growing often appeals to those who value control above all else. In a well-built indoor grow room or tent, you get to dictate nearly every environmental factor — light cycles, temperature, humidity, airflow, and even CO2 levels. This level of customization lets growers push their plants to perform consistently, regardless of the weather outside. It also means you can grow year-round. For someone living in a region with harsh winters or short growing seasons, indoor cultivation can be a game changer. However, this control usually comes at the cost of higher electricity bills, equipment investment, and a steeper learning curve.

Outdoor growing, by contrast, taps into nature's own generosity. When you grow outdoors, your plants soak up sunlight, fresh air, and natural rainfall, which all contribute to healthy, vigorous growth. This method typically demands less upfront cost since you're not relying on artificial lighting or climate systems. Plus, many growers appreciate the satisfaction of tending to cannabis in a natural setting, watching plants stretch and thrive under open skies. But, this freedom also means you're at the mercy of environmental conditions and seasonal timing. Sudden weather changes, pests, and wildlife can complicate the process, which requires some adaptability and resilience from the grower.

One key difference between these two styles lies in the microenvironment each provides. Indoors, you can craft highly specific conditions tailored to the strain's needs, adjusting humidity, temp, and light intensity to encourage optimal growth phases. Outside, the environment fluctuates daily, even hourly, and your plants develop in a more dynamic setting. Some cannabis strains respond beautifully to outdoor conditions, even producing larger buds thanks to full-spectrum sunlight. Meanwhile, other strains flourish with gentle, steady indoor lighting. Choosing your grow style often means matching your preferred cannabis varieties to the environment that suits them best.

Security and privacy are other important factors to weigh. Indoor growing grants discreet cultivation since your plants are hidden away from public view. This can be a major consideration depending on local laws, personal preference, or neighborhood dynamics. Outdoor growing, while absolutely possible in private gardens or gated yards, introduces risks around visibility. A plant's distinctive shape and aroma might attract unwanted attention, calling for extra steps like fences, camouflage, or odor control measures.

Space availability also shapes the decision. If you have ample yard space or access to a rural property, outdoor growing lets you scale easily without the constraints of room dimensions or ventilation concerns. Indoor growers, especially in urban areas or apartments, face spatial limitations that require strategic use of vertical height or tiered shelving to maximize the number of plants. That said, modern indoor setups can be surprisingly compact and efficient, especially with advances in LED lighting and climate tech.

While outdoor cultivation relies heavily on the local climate, indoor cultivation creates its own climate bubble. This advantage lets you dodge problems like unexpected frosts, extreme heatwaves, or heavy rains that can stunt or even kill crops outside. On the flip side, outdoor cannabis benefits from natural sunlight, which covers the full light spectrum. This can promote robust growth and trichome production in a way that artificial lighting may struggle to replicate perfectly, despite technological innovations. Some expert growers even swear by a hybrid approach, starting seedlings indoors before transplanting them outdoors once conditions warm up.

Nutrient delivery also varies between the two styles. Outdoor growers often work with native soil, amended with organic matter or supplements, which feeds plants over longer periods in a natural ecosystem. Indoor growers typically rely on carefully formulated soilless mediums or hydroponic systems, which allow precise nutrient control but require vigilant monitoring and adjustment. Both methods can yield bountiful harvests when managed well, but they demand different skill sets and levels of involvement.

Time commitment can differ as well. Outdoor growing tends to be more seasonal and sometimes lower maintenance during growth phases because much of the environmental management happens naturally. Once plants are in the ground and healthy, you might spend less time tinkering with lights or ventilation. Indoor growing, though more labor-intensive upfront with setup and tuning, allows cultivation throughout all four seasons. Thus, if you want to have multiple harvests a year, indoor might be your best bet.

For beginners, indoor growing might feel overwhelming initially due to all the equipment and tech choices. However, it also offers a more forgiving, contained environment where you can learn basic plant care without uncertainty about unpredictable weather. Outdoor planting offers direct interaction with nature and can be incredibly rewarding, but it exposes growers to external variables that can make it tricky to troubleshoot problems early on. Novices often benefit from starting in a small indoor setup or controlled greenhouse space where factors can be managed more easily.

In the end, both indoor and outdoor growing have stood the test of time as effective cannabis cultivation methods. Your choice will depend on personal circumstances like budget, space, the local environment, desired harvest frequency, and patience level. Neither method is inherently superior—rather, each has unique advantages that can suit different growers and goals. While the chapters ahead will delve deeper into setting up your ideal grow environment and selecting gear, this overview gives you the foundational perspective needed to decide the direction that's right for you.

Keep in mind that flexibility is key. Many cultivators evolve their techniques over time, experimenting with indoor, outdoor, or hybrid growing to find what truly fits their lifestyle and produces the best results. Whatever path you choose, cultivating cannabis at home is an engaging journey. Having a solid grasp of the indoor vs. outdoor landscape lays the groundwork for success as you move forward.

Pros and Cons of Indoor and Outdoor Methods

When it comes to choosing how you want to grow cannabis, deciding between indoor and outdoor methods is one of the biggest crossroads you'll face. Each approach offers unique advantages and drawbacks, shaping how your plants develop, how much control you have, and ultimately, the quality and quantity of your harvest. Understanding these pros and cons upfront can help you pick a style that matches your goals, space, budget, and lifestyle.

Indoor growing is favored by many because it grants you a high degree of control over environmental factors. You can manipulate light, temperature, humidity, and airflow to create ideal conditions, regardless of the season outside. This means you're not bound by weather fluctuations or seasonal daylight changes. For cultivators looking to maximize potency and yield, indoor setups often make that easier.

With indoor grows, one of the biggest advantages is privacy and security. Since the entire grow operation happens inside your home or another enclosed space, it becomes simpler to shield your plants from prying eyes and unwanted visitors. This can also help limit the risk of theft or damage. Additionally, you can start growing at any time of year, as the process is no longer tethered to nature's clock.

However, all this control and privacy come at a cost. Indoor setups require upfront investment in lighting systems, ventilation equipment, grow tents or rooms, and sometimes CO2 supplementation. Electricity bills can spike, too, because of the intense use of lights and fans. Managing heat and humidity indoors demands constant attention, adding to the workload and sometimes stress. Plus, the learning curve is steeper, especially for first-timers who haven't experimented with balancing environmental variables yet.

Outdoor growing, on the other hand, offers a completely different experience. It's cost-effective and naturally sustainable since plants soak up sunlight and rainwater directly. This simplicity appeals to growers on a budget or those just starting out who want to avoid the complexities of electrical setups and artificial lighting. Outdoor gardens often allow your plants to grow larger in size, stretching out roots and branches in open soil, which can result in impressive yields if conditions cooperate.

One of the biggest perks of outdoor cultivation is the way sunlight benefits the plants. Natural solar light contains a full spectrum that's difficult to replicate indoors, which some believe leads to better terpene profiles and more robust growth. The scale can be impressive too—with enough space, outdoor plants can thrive to a size indoor gardens usually can't match. Plus, tending to plants outdoors can feel more connected to nature, offering a rewarding gardening experience beyond just the cannabis itself.

That said, outdoor growing isn't without its risks and limitations. You're at the mercy of weather and pests, both of which can dramatically affect your garden. Sudden cold snaps, heavy rains, or unexpected storms can damage or kill your plants before harvest. Insects, animals, and even neighborhood plants compete for resources and can introduce disease or unwanted pests. Security is another concern: outdoor gardens are more exposed to potential theft or vandalism, which means you might need extra measures like fences, cameras, or strategic location choices.

Another factor outdoor growers need to consider is the growing season, which strictly limits when you can plant and harvest. Unlike indoors, where you might run multiple cycles a year, outdoor cultivation normally follows a single annual timeline tied to daylight hours. This can be a disadvantage if you're aiming for multiple harvests or want more flexibility throughout the year.

While environmental control indoors is a big advantage, it also means managing a complex system that requires experience and commitment. Many growers find themselves troubleshooting ventilation problems, lighting schedules, or humidity issues. The good news is that with practice, these hurdles get easier to tackle, but they're still a significant factor when deciding how to grow.

Conversely, outdoor growing can be more forgiving in some ways. Nature takes care of many factors, but that unpredictability can also be frustrating. You're essentially partnering with the environment, so learning to read weather patterns and adapt your strategies is important. Even so, growing outdoors can be very rewarding for those who appreciate less hands-on micromanagement and more organic growth processes.

From a legal standpoint, some growers find indoor cultivation safer in regions where public visibility of cannabis plants is discouraged or banned. It's easier to keep your operation discreet when it's tucked away inside. Outdoor growing sometimes risks neighbors or passersby noticing your plants, which could raise unwanted questions or complaints if local regulations are strict.

Energy consumption also plays a role in your decision. Indoor grows require more electricity, which not only impacts your wallet but also your environmental footprint. For those who want to grow sustainably, outdoor gardening can be a greener option, although advances in energy-efficient LED lighting are helping reduce indoor energy use.

The choice often boils down to your personal situation. If you have limited space, want fast turnaround times, and don't mind the technical challenges or higher costs, indoor growing could be your best bet. For people with access to secure outdoor space, who prefer a lower-cost and more natural approach, outdoor cultivation might suit them better.

Both growing methods come with learning opportunities. Indoor growers develop skills in environmental control, electrical systems, and precise nutrient management. Outdoor growers become adept at reading natural cues, soil health, and pest prevention in open settings. It's worth considering which skill set appeals to you more, as enjoyment in the process is just as important as the final harvest.

In summary, indoor and outdoor cannabis cultivation methods each offer their own strengths and challenges. Indoor grows shine with control, privacy, and year-round capability but require significant setup and maintenance. Outdoor gardens offer natural light and space with lower operating costs but are vulnerable to environmental unpredictability and security concerns.

Ultimately, the best choice depends on your particular goals, resources, and environment. Many growers even combine both methods—starting plants indoors before moving them outdoors to leverage the benefits of each. Whichever path you choose, understanding these pros and cons will empower you to make informed decisions and set yourself up for success.

Which Growing Method Fits Your Needs?

Choosing the right growing method is one of the most important decisions you'll make when starting your cannabis cultivation journey. It affects everything—from the quality of your harvest to how much time and money you'll invest. Understanding the options and weighing their benefits against your personal situation will save you plenty of headaches down the road. Instead of diving into the technical details, this section focuses on helping you figure out which method aligns best with your lifestyle, goals, and growing environment.

At a high level, cannabis grows either indoors or outdoors, with each having its own subset of approaches and techniques. Neither is inherently better; it all depends on what you're aiming for. Maybe you have limited space and want more control, which usually points to indoor growing. Or maybe you have a backyard and want to maximize natural sunlight, which makes outdoor growing a strong contender. Some growers even use a hybrid approach, combining both methods. What's critical is understanding your priorities and constraints first—then matching those with the method that best suits you.

Indoor grows offer incredible control. You can manage everything from lighting and humidity to temperature and airflow. This control translates to consistent, year-round cultivation on your timetable. If you value predictability and want to fine-tune your environment to get the absolute best out of your plants, indoors might be the way to go. It can feel more like a science experiment, letting you tweak variables and experiment with different strains or growing techniques. But with that control comes higher upfront costs and energy usage—you'll need equipment such as grow lights, ventilation systems, and sometimes even odor control devices.

On the flip side, outdoor growing taps into nature's power. It's generally cheaper since sunlight is free and natural airflow helps manage humidity and temperature.

Outdoor cannabis plants often grow larger due to the unrestricted space and full-spectrum sunlight, which can lead to bigger yields. It's a great option if you have suitable outdoor space and the climate to support it. However, growing outside means dealing with variables you can't fully control—weather, pests, wildlife, and potential legal exposure if privacy is a concern. Outdoor growing tends to be more seasonal, and your success depends heavily on your region's weather patterns.

One factor often overlooked is the amount of time you can dedicate to your grow. Indoor growing demands consistent attention to keep your system balanced, including adjusting lights, watering, and maintaining equipment. Outdoor plants need regular monitoring, especially during rainy or hot spells, but the daily requirements might be less intense. If you're someone who can't check on plants daily or lacks steady time for maintenance, the outdoor method might fit better. Alternatively, investing in automation tools indoors can ease these demands but will increase initial costs.

Security and privacy concerns also play a big role in selecting your method. Growing indoors allows you to keep your operation out of sight, which can be crucial depending on local regulations or shared living arrangements. Outdoor grows, while potentially more challenging to secure from prying eyes or animals, can be less conspicuous if placed properly and well-camouflaged. Always consider your legal environment before deciding. Staying compliant is essential, and your choice should reflect how well you can safeguard your grow from theft, damage, or legal trouble.

Budget is often what brings growers to a crossroads between indoor and outdoor cultivation. Think beyond just the initial cost of seeds or clones. Indoor growing involves a variety of expenses such as lights, fans, fertilizers, filtration systems, and electricity bills that can add up quickly. Outdoor growing, in contrast, tends to have lower overhead. Yet, don't underestimate outdoor costs. You may need fencing, soil amendments, pest control, or protective covers. Plus, unexpected losses from weather or pests can spike costs or reduce your yield, impacting your return on investment.

The type of cannabis you want to grow might also guide your choice. Some strains perform better indoors where conditions are ideal, allowing exotic varieties to thrive and express their unique genetics fully. Others may be more rugged and flourish outdoors, demonstrating resilience against local weather challenges with minimal inputs. If you want to experiment with rare or highly cultivated strains, indoor setups offer a perfect testing ground to dial in their needs without compromise. On the other hand, heirlooms or landrace strains native to your climate can surprise you outdoors with hardiness and abundant growth.

Another consideration is space availability. Indoor growers need a designated area with enough room for lights, plants, and airflow. Some start in small closets, others convert entire rooms, depending on volume desires. Don't overlook height either—taller plants quickly outgrow cramped quarters. Outdoors, you often have more vertical and horizontal freedom, though neighbors, fencing, and local plant limits might restrict how large or numerous your plants can get. Evaluating your physical space honestly fosters realistic plans and prevents frustration.

Climate and weather bring yet another layer of complexity. If you live in a region with harsh winters, short growing seasons, or extended rainy periods, outdoor growing becomes more challenging unless you can provide protective coverings or greenhouses. Indoor grows bypass this limitation completely, creating a controlled bubble that shields plants from harsh elements. But regions blessed with steady sunshine and favorable temperatures often see phenomenal results with outdoor cultivation, reaping natural benefits that artificial lighting tries hard to mimic. Consider the microclimate of your exact location and how much effort you're willing to invest to overcome climate hurdles.

Lastly, personal preference and your ultimate goals matter a lot. Are you growing simply for fun and learning? Maybe a modest outdoor garden suits you well. Are you chasing highly refined, medical-grade flower? Then an indoor grow with precise environmental controls could be a better bet. If maximizing yield is your priority and you want to scale eventually, the path you take now influences your future options. Align your growing style with long-term ambitions so this first step supports everything else going forward.

In summary, the question "Which growing method fits your needs?" boils down to balancing control versus natural advantage, startup investment against ongoing maintenance, and your unique circumstances and goals. Indoor growing offers unmatched control and quality consistency but comes with cost and time commitments. Outdoor growing lets you capitalize on free sunlight and space but introduces unpredictability and seasonality. Many growers find success with mixed approaches, starting outdoors and moving some efforts inside or vice versa.

Understanding your priorities upfront—whether that's budget, space, time, security, or quality—helps create a grow plan that's tailored to you. This foundation will allow you to build confidence in your cannabis cultivation, setting the stage for healthy plants and satisfying harvests. Keep these factors in mind as you explore the specifics of each method in upcoming chapters, and you'll be well on your way to selecting a grow style that truly fits your needs.

CHAPTER 3
ESSENTIAL GROW EQUIPMENT

Now that you've decided on your growing style, it's time to get familiar with the core gear that'll make your cannabis cultivation successful. Whether you're growing indoors or outdoors, having the right equipment—like reliable lighting, quality grow tents, effective fans, and proper filters—can dramatically improve your plant's environment and overall health. It's equally important to pick the right containers and soil that suit your plants' needs along with the nutrients to keep them thriving. You don't have to break the bank to start; plenty of growers find great success with budget-friendly setups that cover the essentials, while those ready to invest can explore premium options that offer advanced features and durability. This chapter sets you up with the foundational tools bridging your growing knowledge to a flourishing crop.

Lights, Tents, Fans, and Filters for Growing

When setting up an indoor cannabis garden, few things matter as much as the core gear—lights, tents, fans, and filters. Together, they create the foundation for a healthy, productive grow space. Each piece plays a vital role in replicating the ideal environment for your plants, and getting them right from the start is essential to avoid costly mistakes later. Whether you're just starting or looking to improve your current setup, understanding how these components work together will empower you to cultivate better buds with less hassle.

Let's begin with lighting because it's often the heartbeat of any indoor garden. Cannabis is a light-hungry plant that thrives under specific spectrums and intensities. Your choice of lights influences everything from vegetative growth to flowering and bud development. You want a system that delivers not only enough brightness but also the right quality of light to mimic the sun's natural rhythms. A strong, evenly distributed light source encourages robust, uniform plant growth, preventing weak spots and stretching that can occur under poor lighting.

Beyond just brightness, heat output from lights is another factor you can't ignore. While high-intensity discharge (HID) lights like HPS and MH have been trusted staples for years, they can run hot, raising the temperature in your grow room dangerously if not paired with adequate ventilation. On the other hand, LEDs have become popular for their energy efficiency and reduced heat output, allowing you to keep plants closer without fear of burns or heat stress. Choosing between these options mostly depends on your budget, grow space size, and personal preferences—but whichever you pick, it must be balanced with effective air circulation.

Now, onto grow tents. These are game-changers for indoor growers, creating a controlled micro-environment that's easy to manage and maximizes your gear's efficiency. A good quality grow tent keeps light where it belongs—inside—so your cannabis plants soak up every photon of energy. Plus, tents protect your garden from outside contamination like pests and dust, while also helping to regulate humidity and temperature. The reflective interior walls boost the power of your grow lights by bouncing light around, ensuring even coverage for all plants in the tent.

When picking a tent, size is everything. Bigger isn't always better if you don't have the space or time to maintain a larger number of plants. Think carefully about how many plants you plan to grow and how much room they'll need to develop fully. A cramped tent can lead to overcrowding, poor airflow, and increased risk of disease. On the flip side, a tent that's too large might waste electricity and make it harder to maintain stable environmental conditions. It's smart to start with a tent size that fits your goals and expand as you gain experience.

Ventilation is the unsung hero in your grow room. Fans and filters work in tandem to keep the air moving, maintain temperature, and prevent humidity buildup. Without proper airflow, your garden might turn into a hotspot for mold, mildew, and pests. Good ventilation also strengthens stems by simulating outdoor breezes, resulting in sturdier plants ready to support heavier buds. You'll typically need both intake and exhaust fans to pull fresh air in while expelling stale, oxygen-depleted air out.

One tricky part of ventilation is managing odors—a big issue for many growers. Cannabis plants release strong smells, especially during flowering, so having a high-quality carbon filter in your ventilation system can help neutralize these odors before they escape your grow space. Carbon filters trap scent particles, keeping your grow discreet and your home smelling fresh. When selecting a filter, consider the size of your tent and airflow rate of your fans to ensure the system runs smoothly without causing negative air pressure or restricting airflow.

Fan size and placement deserve thought as well. Oscillating fans positioned inside your tent help break up stagnant pockets of air, moving it gently across leaves and around plants. This circulation reduces hot spots and prevents moisture from settling on surfaces where mold could thrive. For exhaust fans, ducting is important—using insulated, flexible ducting helps reduce noise and guides air efficiently outside your grow area. It's also wise to include a fan speed controller, so you can fine-tune airflow depending on the weather or growth stage.

One practical advantage of grow tents is how readily they integrate with other equipment. You can easily hang your lights, mount fans, and secure filters at ideal heights to maximize efficiency. Most tents come with built-in straps, ports for fans and ducting, and sturdy frames designed to hold heavier gear safely. This convenience accelerates setup time and makes adjustments easier as your grow evolves. Plus, tents keep dust and other contaminants at bay, which is especially helpful in urban areas or dusty homes.

It's worth mentioning that while each component matters, their real power lies in how well they work together. A powerful light without proper ventilation risks cooking your plants or drying them out. A well-ventilated tent with inadequate lighting won't produce the dense flowers you're after. And an odor control system that's too small won't effectively mask strong flower smells. Take the time to match your equipment's capacity and performance to your grow space size and plant count, so every piece supports the others seamlessly.

The good news is there's an equipment option for any budget. Entry-level kits bundle lights, tents, and ventilation gear at reasonable prices, making them perfect for beginners testing the waters. They might not pack the punch of premium systems, but they're a solid place to start. For those aiming to scale up or dial in precision, investing in top-tier LEDs, commercial-grade tents, and whisper-quiet inline fans and filters is worth every penny. The payoff is healthier plants, less stress managing the environment, and ultimately, a more satisfying harvest.

Beyond gear specifics, keep in mind the importance of maintenance. Regularly clean your fans and filters to prevent buildup that could clog airflow. Check tent seals and zippers to avoid light leaks or pests sneaking in. Routinely inspect your lighting to catch flickering bulbs or failing components early. A little upkeep goes a long way in keeping your grow environment stable and your plants thriving.

In summary, lights, tents, fans, and filters are your frontline tools in shaping a cannabis grow space that supports vibrant growth and impressive yields. They create a controlled habitat that simulates the natural world while letting you tailor conditions to your plants' needs. Mastering this equipment lays the groundwork for every other part of successful cultivation, from choosing the right seeds to timing your harvest. With the right setup, you're setting yourself up for a rewarding growing journey that combines science, art, and a little bit of patience.

Selecting the Right Pots, Soil, and Nutrients

Once you've got your grow space set up with proper lighting and ventilation, the next big step is choosing the right pots, soil, and nutrients. These are the foundation for healthy cannabis plants and can make or break your entire grow operation. Every detail counts—from the size of the pot to the composition of the soil and the nutrient blend you use. Understanding these essentials will help you unlock your plants' true potential.

Let's start with pots. There's a surprising variety available, and the choice affects root development, water retention, and even airflow. Plastic pots are the most common and budget-friendly, but they might not offer the best drainage or air circulation for your plants. Fabric pots, often called smart pots or air pots, have breathable sides that encourage roots to air prune themselves. This results in a denser and healthier root system, improving nutrient uptake and overall vigor. If you're someone who prefers to reuse pots across grows, plastic can be durable, but fabric pots are typically lightweight and easy to store when not in use.

Container size matters too. Smaller pots are easier to manage but limit how large your plants can grow before becoming root-bound. A general rule is to start with 1-3 gallon pots for seedlings and young plants, then transplant them into 5-gallon or larger containers for their flowering stage. Larger pots hold more soil and retain moisture longer, which can reduce watering frequency, but also weigh more and require more floor space. Keep your grow space constraints in mind while making your decision.

Drainage is non-negotiable. No matter what pot type you choose, make sure it has adequate holes at the bottom to prevent waterlogging. Standing water is a silent killer that drowns roots and promotes fungal growth. Some growers add a layer of perlite, gravel, or hydroton at the bottom of their pots to further improve drainage and prevent root rot. These small steps can save you from major headaches down the line.

Moving on to soil—this is where the magic really starts. Cannabis thrives in a well-draining, nutrient-rich medium that allows roots to stretch and breathe. The composition of your soil depends on whether you want to go organic or use a more controlled synthetic nutrient approach. Organic soils often include components like compost, worm castings, peat moss, coco coir, and various amendments such as bone meal or kelp meal. These ingredients provide a slow-release food source for your plants and encourage beneficial microbial activity, which in turn helps with nutrient uptake and disease resistance.

If you want quick results and greater control over feeding, soilless mixes or hydroponic substrates might be the way to go. Peat-based mixes or coco coir blends offer a clean, inert medium that doesn't supply nutrients on its own but allows you to tailor your feed precisely. This flexibility is great once you gain experience because you can customize nutrient concentrations for each growth phase. Just remember, soilless mediums demand more attention to watering schedules and pH management since there's less natural buffering capacity compared to organic soils.

Another important soil factor is pH. Cannabis favors slightly acidic conditions, with an ideal pH range of 6.0 to 7.0 for soil grows. Outside this window, nutrient availability drops, and your plants may show signs of deficiencies even if nutrients are present. Testing your soil's pH regularly with a pH meter or test kit is a simple practice that pays huge dividends. Adjusting pH can be done with additives like dolomite lime in soil or pH up/down solutions in liquid feeds.

Once you've selected the right pots and soil, nutrition becomes your best weapon for vigorous growth and bountiful harvests. Cannabis requires a balanced diet of macronutrients—nitrogen (N), phosphorus (P), and potassium (K)—alongside micronutrients like calcium, magnesium, and iron. The key is recognizing which nutrients your plants need at each stage and supplying them accordingly. Overfeeding can burn roots and stunt growth, while underfeeding leaves plants weak and vulnerable.

For soil grows, many beginners start with a pre-fertilized soil mix that contains enough nutrients for the seedling and vegetative stages. This allows you to water with plain pH-balanced water for the first several weeks, reducing the risk of nutrient burn. As plants mature and enter the flowering phase, supplemental feeding with organic or synthetic fertilizers is usually necessary to meet their increased demands.

Organic nutrient sources are popular because they tend to release slowly and enhance soil biology. Typical options include bat guano, fish emulsion, seaweed extract, and compost teas. These inputs not only feed the plants but also nurture beneficial microbes in the root zone, fostering a natural and resilient growing environment. If you prefer a hands-off approach, many commercial organic nutrient lines are available and formulated specifically for cannabis.

Synthetic nutrients, on the other hand, deliver precise amounts of each element, absorbed quickly by the plants. They're often used in hydroponics or when growers want to push growth aggressively. Keep in mind, synthetic nutrients require careful monitoring of solution pH and electrical conductivity (EC) to prevent toxicity or deficiencies. Beginners may find synthetic feeding more complex initially, but with practice, it's a powerful tool for maximizing yields.

Water quality also plays an integral role in nutrient availability. Tap water varies widely in mineral content and chlorine levels, both of which can affect nutrient uptake and microbial life in the soil. Many growers opt for filtered or distilled water, or at least let tap water sit out for 24 hours to allow chlorine to dissipate. Knowing your water's baseline helps you adjust nutrient formulations properly and avoid unwanted surprises.

One overlooked factor when selecting pots, soil, and nutrients is environmental compatibility. Your grow space's temperature, humidity, and airflow will influence how fast your soil dries out and how nutrients behave. In hotter environments, lighter soils with good aeration reduce the risk of root heat stress, while cooler conditions might require soil with higher water retention. Pay attention to these subtle details to keep your roots comfortable, ultimately leading to healthier, more resilient plants.

To sum it up, there's no one-size-fits-all answer when it comes to choosing pots, soil, and nutrients. However, understanding the relationship between these elements and the unique needs of cannabis plants will guide you in crafting a grow medium that supports vigorous growth from seedling to harvest. Start with breathable pots sized to suit your plants, choose a soil or medium that matches your level of experience and feeding preferences, and provide balanced, phase-appropriate nutrients. Your plants will reward you with robust health and excellent yields when these fundamentals are dialed in.

Keep in mind that the learning curve can be smooth if you test and observe closely. Don't hesitate to experiment with small changes in soil mixes or nutrient ratios over successive grows to find what truly works best in your environment. This process of fine-tuning is where many successful growers separate themselves from those who struggle. The right combination of pot, soil, and nutrients forms the rock-solid foundation upon which all other growing techniques rest.

Budget Versus Premium Equipment Setups

When it comes to setting up your cannabis grow, one of the first big decisions you'll face is whether to go with a budget setup or invest in premium equipment. Both approaches have their merits, and understanding the differences can help you make smarter choices that fit your goals and wallet. Of course, a higher price tag doesn't always guarantee success, nor does a frugal approach mean you can't produce quality buds. The trick lies in knowing which pieces of equipment matter most and where you can compromise without sacrificing your crop's health or yield.

For beginners or growers just testing the waters, budget setups offer a low-risk entry into the world of indoor cannabis cultivation. These kits are often compact, user-friendly, and come with all the basics needed to get started. Typically, they include an affordable grow tent, basic LED or fluorescent lighting, a simple ventilation system, and starter pots or trays. Because the upfront costs are modest, they allow you to learn the essential mechanics—like maintaining temperature, humidity, and light cycles—without the pressure of heavy financial investment.

However, budget gear often means compromises. The lighting may be less intense or less tailored to the precise needs of cannabis at different growth phases, which can impact plant development and final potency. Ventilation systems might be smaller or less efficient, increasing risks related to stale air or heat buildup. Also, cheaper grow tents may have less durable materials or fewer reflective surfaces, which can reduce overall light effectiveness. This doesn't mean low-budget setups can't yield decent results, but patience and some clever adjustments become key factors in overcoming those limits.

On the other end of the spectrum, premium equipment is designed to provide optimal growing conditions right out of the box. High-end grow lights, such as full-spectrum LEDs or ceramic metal halide (CMH) lamps, deliver tailored light spectrums that closely mimic natural sunlight, encouraging vigorous growth and maximizing cannabinoid production. These lights come with adjustable intensity features, better energy efficiency, and longer lifespans. The initial cost is steeper, but many growers find that the performance and reliability justify the investment.

Premium tents also step up in quality, constructed from heavier-duty materials with excellent light-proof seals and highly reflective interiors. These features improve light penetration and prevent light leaks that could disrupt your plants' photoperiod. Ventilation equipment in premium setups often includes quiet, powerful inline fans combined with high-quality carbon filters, which not only control temperature and humidity better but also actively reduce odors. This level of environmental control can make all the difference, especially for growers who want to cultivate discreetly or in limited spaces.

Another key difference lies in automation and monitoring. Budget systems tend to rely on manual adjustments—checking temperatures, humidity, and light timers daily—while premium setups might include integrated digital controllers, sensors, and smart plugs that automate many tasks. These tools not only save you time but also reduce human error, which can be vital to maintaining consistent and ideal conditions throughout the grow.

Despite these contrasts, it's important to realize that success isn't dictated solely by the equipment you buy. Grower knowledge, attentiveness, and problem-solving skills consistently play a larger role in achieving a bountiful harvest. That's why newcomers often succeed with budget setups if they learn to optimize airflow, use supplemental reflectors to maximize light, and carefully monitor their grow environment. Conversely, premium equipment can still be underutilized if the grower neglects regular maintenance or fails to understand how to fine-tune their system.

One practical approach many growers take is to start with a modest, budget-conscious setup focused on learning the ropes. As confidence builds and specific needs become clearer, they gradually upgrade key components such as lighting or ventilation. This incremental investment reduces the initial financial burden while targeting improvements where they will have the most impact. For example, swapping out a basic LED for a high-quality full-spectrum fixture often yields noticeable gains in growth rate and bud quality without overhauling the entire system.

It's also worth considering the scale and goals of your grow. If you plan to cultivate just a few plants for personal use, a budget setup might easily meet your needs. In contrast, growers pursuing larger yields or aiming to produce top-shelf cannabis may find that premium equipment provides better control over subtle environmental factors that push plants to their full potential. This is especially relevant when striving for specific cannabinoid profiles or terpene-rich aromas where consistent, precise conditions are crucial.

Energy consumption is another factor feeding into the budget versus premium decision. While cheaper lights might have lower upfront costs, they tend to be less energy-efficient, meaning your electricity bills could rise significantly over time. Premium systems often feature energy-saving technologies and better heat management that translate into lower operational costs, balancing their initial expense. For growers facing strict household budgets, this operational efficiency can be a meaningful consideration.

Maintenance and durability differ markedly, too. Budget gear frequently involves more trial and error, as components may wear out or perform inconsistently over multiple grows. Premium equipment is typically crafted to last longer under the high demands of indoor cultivation and may come with better customer support or warranties. This peace of mind can prove invaluable, particularly for first-time growers who might be intimidated by technical troubleshooting.

Beyond the equipment, your personal comfort and work experience matter. Premium setups often feature ergonomic benefits like easy-access panels, noise-reducing ventilation, and superior light coverage that make daily tending less cumbersome and more enjoyable. The physical ease of managing your grow can positively affect how frequently you check on your plants and how quickly you respond to environmental shifts.

Before deciding which route to take, consider the local legal framework and your privacy needs as well. Premium gear with top-notch odor control and sound dampening can be critical for growers in sensitive or urban areas. Meanwhile, budget setups might require additional DIY modifications to manage smells or noise, which adds complexity but can still be done if you're resourceful.

Ultimately, there's no one-size-fits-all answer when choosing between budget and premium growing equipment. The ideal setup balances your available funds, your commitment to the craft, and your desired outcomes. Starting small and learning as you go builds invaluable experience without breaking the bank, while selective investments in premium components can elevate your results when you're ready. Whichever path you choose, staying focused on consistent environmental conditions and attentive plant care will always be the foundation for cultivating healthy, potent cannabis.

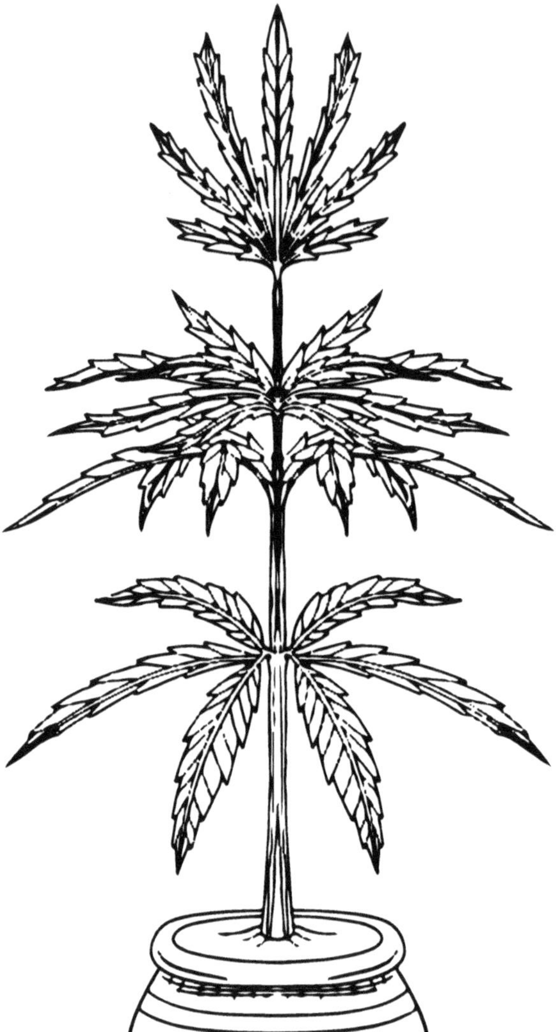

Chapter 4
Picking the Right Seeds

Choosing the right seeds is the foundation of any successful cannabis grow, and it sets the stage for the entire cultivation journey. Whether you're starting fresh or looking to refine your crop, understanding the different seed types and where to source quality genetics matters more than you might think. Feminized seeds eliminate the guesswork by producing only female plants, which means less effort and no surprises with unwanted males, while autoflower seeds offer a faster, more hands-off approach that's perfect for growers wanting to cut down on wait times without sacrificing yield. Regular seeds, though a bit trickier because of their mixed genders, remain popular for breeders and those interested in preserving genetic diversity. The seed you pick should reflect your growing goals, experience level, and patience, but it's just as important to trust reputable seed banks that provide tested, stable genetics—something you'll appreciate when your plants start to flourish. In short, investing time now in choosing the right seeds pays off in more robust plants, better harvests, and a more rewarding growing experience overall.

Feminized, Autoflower, and Regular Seeds Compared

Choosing the right type of cannabis seeds is one of the most important decisions you'll make before starting your grow. The main categories to know about are feminized, autoflower, and regular seeds—each comes with its unique characteristics, advantages, and challenges. Understanding how they differ can help you pick seeds that fit your experience level, growing environment, and final goals.

Let's start with feminized seeds, which have become the go-to choice for many growers, especially beginners and those who want the most straightforward growing experience. These seeds are bred specifically to produce female plants almost exclusively. Since only female cannabis plants produce buds, feminized seeds eliminate the unpredictability of male plants popping up and potentially pollinating your crop, which would reduce bud quality. Growing feminized seeds means you can focus all your energy on cultivating potent, flower-producing plants without having to identify and remove males during the grow.

One of the biggest benefits of feminized seeds is consistency. Because they're engineered to be female, you can expect a higher success rate of quality flowering plants per seed, making them ideal for home growers, especially if space, time, or resources are limited. They're pretty much the industry standard now, found in most seed banks and come from stabilized genetics.

However, while feminized seeds remove the risk of unwanted males, they might not be the best fit if you want to breed your own plants or experiment with genetics. That's where regular seeds come in. Regular seeds are what nature produces, containing about a 50/50 split of male and female plants. For growers looking to clone or create new strains, regular seeds are essential because you need male plants for pollination and breeding.

Growing regular seeds requires a bit more effort because you have to identify and cull male plants early to avoid pollination, which can be stressful and time-consuming, especially for beginners. But for those interested in preserving and manipulating genetics, regular seeds offer more flexibility and control. Plus, some purists believe the plants from regular seeds grow more vigorously and with better natural vigor than feminized plants, although this can vary.

Then there are autoflower seeds, which have changed the game in recent years by integrating genetics from Cannabis ruderalis, a hardy strain known for automatic flowering. Unlike feminized or regular seeds derived mainly from photoperiod plants, autoflowers don't rely on light cycles to initiate flowering. Instead, they flower on a fixed timeline regardless of light exposure, typically completing their full life cycle—from seed to harvest—in as little as 8 to 12 weeks.

This unique trait makes autoflower seeds incredibly appealing, especially for growers dealing with limited space, outdoor growers with shorter growing seasons, or anyone wanting quick turnaround times between harvests. Because autoflowers initiate flowering automatically at a certain age, you don't have to fuss with changing light schedules or worry about when to trigger the flowering phase.

But autoflowers aren't perfect. Historically, they tended to have smaller yields and lower potency compared to photoperiod plants. Advances in breeding have lessened this gap significantly, but yields might still be smaller than what you'd get from feminized photoperiod seeds under the right conditions. Another consideration is that autoflowers generally have shorter vegetative phases, limiting the amount of training or pruning you can do to maximize yields. If maximizing flower size and quality is your goal, autoflowers might require a different approach than traditional seeds.

On the plus side, autoflowers often display incredible resilience to environmental stressors and pests, partly thanks to their ruderalis heritage. Many growers find them easier to manage, especially when growing outdoors in areas with unpredictable weather or light schedules that don't favor photoperiod plants. Also, autoflowers usually don't grow as tall or wide, which can be a benefit in small growing spaces.

In terms of seed cost, regular seeds are often the cheapest option, followed by feminized seeds, with autoflower seeds usually commanding the highest prices due to their specialized breeding. It's worth considering that while autoflower seeds cost more upfront, the quick turnaround and potential for multiple harvests per season can balance the economics out, depending on your growing goals.

From a beginner's standpoint, feminized seeds offer an excellent balance of ease and yield without the need to identify males, making them the most popular choice for first-time growers. Autoflowers, while super easy to grow and quick to harvest, might require a learning curve to optimize their unique life cycle. Regular seeds, though more challenging for novices due to the sexing process, provide unmatched genetic diversity and breeding opportunities for those who want to dive deeper into cannabis cultivation.

Another factor to keep in mind is the grow environment and lifestyle. If you're growing indoors with the ability to control light cycles, feminized photoperiod seeds give you maximum control over growth stages and plant training, meaning you can manipulate the light to keep plants in the vegetative phase as long as you want. Autoflowers, tied to their internal clock, limit that control but offer simplicity. Outdoors, autoflowers might be your best bet in northern climates with short seasons, while feminized seeds shine in more temperate zones where longer flowering cycles are feasible.

Finally, seed choice can impact the overall experience and satisfaction of your grow. While genetics matter a lot, the seed type influences how you manage the plants, the schedule you follow, and ultimately, the enjoyment of the cultivation process. Knowing the differences between feminized, autoflower, and regular seeds arms you with the knowledge to match plants to your goals, skill level, and environment, setting you up for a successful harvest.

When deciding among these seed types, consider what matters most to you: ease and predictability, speed and resilience, or genetic exploration and breeding potential. Each seed type plays a unique role in the cannabis growing landscape, and understanding their strengths and limitations will help you grow smarter, not just harder.

Where to Buy Quality Cannabis Seeds

Now that you understand the importance of selecting the right seeds for your cannabis cultivation journey, the next crucial step is figuring out where to purchase those seeds. Finding quality cannabis seeds isn't just about grabbing the first pack that pops up in a quick search. Your source influences everything—from genetic stability and germination rates to legal compliance and your ultimate yield. With so many options available, it's worth taking the time to choose reputable sellers who offer real value and trustworthy products.

One of the most popular venues to buy cannabis seeds is licensed seed banks. Seed banks are specialized retailers that maintain a large catalog of genetics from breeders around the world. These professionals rigorously test and store seeds under optimal conditions to ensure quality and viability. Buying from a well-established seed bank gives you the assurance that you're getting authentic strains with clear descriptions of their effects, flowering times, THC/CBD content, and growth characteristics. It's not just about convenience—it's about certainty.

Many seed banks operate online, which has opened up the market tremendously. Online seed banks usually provide detailed strain profiles, customer reviews, and germination guarantees, helping growers—whether new or experienced—make an informed decision. Plus, they typically ship discreetly and securely, which is a significant consideration depending on your location and its regulations. However, the convenience of online shopping doesn't mean you should pick just any web store. Do your homework. Look for transparency regarding their breeding practices, clear return policies, and customer service responsiveness. These factors point to a seed bank that stands behind its product.

Another important avenue to explore is local dispensaries or licensed cannabis retailers, especially in regions where recreational or medicinal cannabis is legal. Some dispensaries stock cannabis seeds from trusted breeders, offering customers a chance to see packages in person before buying. This can be helpful if you prefer face-to-face interaction or need advice tailored to your local climate and cultivation environment. Staff at knowledgeable dispensaries often have first-hand growing experience and can recommend strains that suit your skill level and desired effects.

While local seed shops and dispensaries might seem like the safest bet, they sometimes have limited strain selections compared to large seed banks. Still, for beginners, the direct support can make a big difference in starting out on the right foot. It's also an opportunity to connect with fellow growers or join local cannabis communities and clubs. These connections can later provide valuable insights, cut down on trial and error, and enrich your growing experience as a whole.

It's crucial to be cautious about buying cannabis seeds from unverified sources like street dealers or peer-to-peer online marketplaces. The risks include receiving seeds that are old, non-viable, or even counterfeit. The genetic integrity may be compromised, resulting in plants that don't perform as advertised or have lower potency. Additionally, without clear legal channels, you could expose yourself to legal trouble or financial loss if your package is seized or fails to arrive. In short, saving a few bucks upfront is rarely worth the potential headaches and disappointments.

One method to check a seed bank's credibility—especially online—is to seek out grower forums, review sites, and independent grow journals where users share their planting results and shopping experiences. Genuine buyers often post photos of their harvests and detailed notes about seed quality and germination success. A seed bank with a consistent history of positive feedback is typically a reliable choice. You might even find tips for exclusive promotions or new strain releases that haven't hit bigger markets yet.

Many well-known seed banks also offer specialized seeds such as feminized, autoflowering, and regular seeds. The availability of these options allows you to pick a product aligned with your growing goals and conditions, but make sure you confirm what exactly is included in your purchase. Some sellers provide sample packs or trial options if you want to experiment with different genetics without committing to large quantities. This can be a smart approach to learn which varieties thrive under your particular care regimen.

International shipping is another factor to consider but depends heavily on local laws regarding cannabis seeds. Seed banks located in countries with established cannabis laws often ship worldwide, but customs and import restrictions vary. It's a good idea to verify whether importing seeds into your state or country is legal and what precautions the seed bank uses to ensure your order passes through without issue. Some sellers use discreet packaging or offer free replacement guarantees if your shipment is confiscated. These policies provide a safety net, especially for first-time buyers wary of running into legal snags.

For growers aiming to elevate their cultivation to the next level, investing in genetics from well-known breeders and seed banks renowned for quality is essential. These breeders spend years stabilizing strains and developing hybrids that produce consistent, robust plants with desirable traits. When you buy seeds from a trusted breeder, you're not just purchasing a product—you're buying into expertise and a track record of success. This reliability can mean the difference between frustration and a flourishing grow.

At the same time, emerging breeders and boutique seed companies are rapidly gaining respect in the grower community. These smaller operations often focus on unique, rare, or heirloom cannabis strains that deliver distinctive flavors, aromas, and effects. If you're someone who enjoys experimenting and diversifying your garden, sourcing seeds from these breeders can add excitement and variety. Just make sure the issuer has good references and, if possible, customer guarantees to back up their claims about seed quality.

Remember that no matter where you buy your cannabis seeds, quality control starts with you. Always review the seed descriptions carefully before purchasing. Look for packs that clearly state germination rates, seed maturity, and any certifications or awards the strain has received. Packaging should be sturdy to protect seeds from light, humidity, and damage during transit. Sometimes seed companies include growing tips or detailed instructions that can help you get the most out of your genetics right from the start.

One final note is to stay up to date with changes in cannabis laws that could affect seed purchasing. The legal landscape is evolving rapidly in many places, bringing fresh opportunities but also new requirements. Some states or countries now allow growers to buy directly from licensed producers or seed banks, while others maintain restrictions on certain seed types. Staying informed helps you avoid unintentional missteps and assures a smooth, legal start to your home cannabis cultivation.

In summary, the options for purchasing cannabis seeds are numerous, but quality, reliability, and legality must be your guiding principles. Licensed seed banks—whether online or local—offer the best combination of genetics, customer support, and legal compliance. Dispensaries can provide personalized advice and immediate access but may have limited strains. Be wary of untrustworthy or informal sellers to protect your investment and growing success. With the right source, you're setting your cultivation journey up for a strong, productive foundation.

Germination Methods That Produce Results

Once you've chosen the right cannabis seeds, the next critical step is germination—the process that kickstarts life for every successful grow. Germination might seem straightforward, but it's actually the foundation that determines how strong and healthy your young plants will be. Without a reliable germination method, even the best seeds might fail, leaving you frustrated and delaying your growing schedule. That's why understanding the methods that consistently produce results is an essential part of picking the right seeds and ensuring they flourish.

One of the most popular and time-tested approaches is the classic paper towel method. This technique is praised for its simplicity and reliability, making it ideal for beginners and experts alike. All you need is a couple of clean paper towels, a plate, and a warm environment. By placing your seeds between damp (but not soaking wet) paper towels, you create a moist environment that mimics spring rains without drowning the seed. This encourages the seed's shell to soften, allowing the taproot to break through. Within a few days, you can usually observe the taproot emerging, a critical sign your seed is alive and ready to be planted.

However, the paper towel method demands careful attention. Dampness must be maintained but not overdone, since too much water can drown the seeds or create a breeding ground for mold. The warmth factor is just as vital—ideally, seeds should remain in temperatures between 70 and 85 degrees Fahrenheit to promote quick germination. Some growers use a heat mat set to low temperatures to maintain this consistent warmth, especially in cooler climates or indoors. Small details like these separate successful germination runs from disappointing failures.

Another highly effective method is direct planting, where seeds are sown straight into the growing medium—usually soil, coco coir, or a starter cube. This method reduces the risk of damaging delicate taproots that sometimes occurs when transferring germinated seeds from paper towels to soil. For those who prefer a "set it and forget it" style, planting directly might suit your workflow better. The seed stays snug in the environment it will grow in, making the transition seamless. However, it requires you to maintain optimal soil moisture and temperature carefully since there's no way to check on seeds without disturbing the soil.

Many growers swear by starting seeds in soilless mediums like rockwool cubes or peat pellets. These substrates offer excellent moisture retention and air circulation, helping delicate roots thrive early on. The advantage here is the easy transplantability—once seedlings have established a healthy root ball, they can be transferred cleanly to pots or hydro systems with minimal shock. While rockwool cubes are more common in hydroponic setups, peat pellets are favored in organic soil grows since they add nutrients without compacting the medium.

Some advanced growers employ water germination, where seeds briefly soak in water for 12 to 24 hours before continuing their development on paper towels or directly for planting. Water soaking softens the seed shell, increasing germination speed. However, this technique carries a risk: extend soaking too long and seeds may rot due to lack of oxygen. Timing is crucial here, so pay close attention if you decide to give this method a try.

Several growers have also experimented with pre-germination seed treatments to boost results. For example, soaking seeds in a mild solution of hydrogen peroxide can sometimes reduce bacterial and fungal growth, effectively sterilizing the seed shell. Others gently nick or scarify the seed coat to help water penetrate more easily. While these options can be useful, they require a delicate touch and some experience—too much can damage the seed, too little might be ineffective.

Regardless of the method you choose, a common thread is the attention to environmental conditions. Light, moisture, temperature, and cleanliness can't be underestimated. Using sterile tools and clean materials drastically cuts down the odds of mold or fungus interfering with your precious seeds. Also, a warm, dark space is preferable since exposure to light before sprouting might disrupt germination. Some growers use small labeled containers or humidity domes to keep conditions ideal and organized, especially when germinating multiple strains simultaneously.

Patience also plays a big role. Although most seeds sprout within three to seven days under good conditions, some take longer. Rushing to plant a seed that hasn't cracked its shell can damage it or give it poor chances of survival. Conversely, leaving seeds waiting too long in a damp environment can cause them to drown or rot, making timing a balancing act. You'll want to monitor without interfering too much—carefully lifting paper towels or gently peeking at your medium without drastic disturbance.

One often overlooked tip is record-keeping. Tracking which methods you used and the germination success rate gives you valuable data for future grows. Over time, you'll refine your preferred techniques and adjust them based on the strains you're working with. Some strains just respond better to certain approaches, so having a grow journal can identify patterns, saving effort and increasing yield quality down the line.

Environmental control during germination is critical because seedlings are delicate and vulnerable in those early days. Freezing temperatures, excessive heat, or poor air circulation can slow or stall the process and increase the chance of failure. A stable, moderate temperature combined with steady humidity around

70% to 80% usually provides the best environment for young cannabis seeds to wake up and send out their first roots.

While it may seem like a minor first step, getting germination right has a ripple effect throughout the entire grow. Healthy seedlings lead to vigorous vegetative growth and better odds of producing big, resin-rich buds later on. Incorrect or careless germination can stunt growth from the start, meaning the extra time, energy, and resources spent later might not pay off.

In short, germination methods that produce results rely on a few simple but vital principles: moisture without drowning, warmth with stability, cleanliness to avoid contamination, and patience to let nature take its course. Whether you choose paper towels, direct planting, or starter plugs, the key is to respect the seed's needs and provide an environment where it can thrive.

With this foundation firmly in place, your cannabis seeds will be more than ready to move confidently into the next stages of growth. The effort invested in mastering germination pays dividends in a healthy, robust crop that makes all the difference come harvest time.

CHAPTER 5
THE VEGETATIVE STAGE

The vegetative stage sets the foundation for a healthy and productive cannabis plant, where rapid growth takes center stage and establishing strong roots, sturdy stems, and lush foliage becomes the priority. During this phase, providing the right balance of light, water, and nutrients is crucial to encourage vigorous development without stressing the plants. This period is all about encouraging leafy growth that will support future buds, so paying close attention to light cycles—usually long daylight hours—and consistent watering while avoiding over-saturation helps ensure robust performance. While the plants stretch and thicken, this is the optimal time to start training techniques that will maximize yields later on, shaping your crop for success. Recognizing signs of healthy growth, including vibrant green leaves and firm stems, will guide your adjustments and keep your plants thriving as they prepare for the next exciting stage of development.

Light Cycles, Watering, and Nutrient Basics

Transitioning into the vegetative stage marks a critical phase in your cannabis plants' development. They're shifting from tiny seedlings to robust young plants, getting ready to build the structure that will support future buds. Getting the fundamentals right—especially light schedules, watering habits, and nutrition—can make all the difference in producing healthy, vigorous plants that set the stage for a successful harvest.

The light cycle during the vegetative stage isn't just about keeping lights on—it's about mimicking natural conditions that signal your plants to grow. Typically, most growers opt for an 18/6 cycle: 18 hours of light followed by 6 hours of complete darkness each day. This extended light period encourages the plant to focus energy on growing leaves, stems, and roots rather than starting to flower. Some growers push for a 24-hour light cycle, especially indoors, believing it maximizes growth. While plants can handle nonstop light during veg, a short dark period often benefits the plant by giving it a rest phase, which can improve overall vigor and reduce stress.

The quality and intensity of light also come into play but won't be detailed extensively here since we'll cover that later. However, it's good to know that cannabis thrives under full-spectrum light resembling sunlight, especially with plenty of blue wavelengths that promote leafy growth during veg. Using the right lighting and avoiding shading or overcrowding ensures each plant soaks in enough energy to keep growing upward and outward effectively.

When it comes to watering, it's a balancing act that many growers find tricky at first. Cannabis plants require a consistent but moderate watering regimen during the vegetative stage—too much can drown roots and invite disease; too little leaves the plant thirsty and stunted. The rule of thumb is to water deeply, soaking the growing medium enough for roots to access moisture thoroughly, then allow the medium to dry out partially before the next watering. This lets the roots breathe and encourages them to spread out searching for water, strengthening the plant's foundation.

Many beginners fall into the trap of overwatering because they see drooping leaves and assume the plant is dehydrated, while in reality, the roots might be suffocating from excess moisture. Always check the weight of your pots or the dryness of the soil a couple of inches down before adding water again. Early-stage plants with smaller root systems will need less frequent watering, and containers with good drainage will help avoid waterlogging problems.

Water quality isn't a minor detail either. Cannabis favors a balanced pH—usually between 6.0 and 7.0 for soil grows—and consistent water chemistry. Using tap water with a high chlorine content or unbalanced pH can slow growth or cause nutrient lockout. For this reason, many growers treat their water by letting it sit overnight to dissipate chlorine or by using pH-test kits and adjustments. Maintaining a steady environment allows your plants to uptake nutrients efficiently and avoid shocking their delicate root systems.

Speaking of nutrients, during the vegetative stage, plants primarily demand macronutrients—nitrogen, phosphorus, and potassium—in different proportions compared to other growth phases. Nitrogen reigns supreme here because it drives leaf and stem development. You want a nutrient formula designed for veg that offers higher nitrogen, moderate phosphorus, and balanced potassium. This encourages lush, vigorous growth without pushing your plants into premature flowering or causing nutrient burn.

Micronutrients such as calcium, magnesium, and iron also play subtle but crucial roles during veg. They support enzymatic functions, cell wall structure, and chlorophyll production. Even if you're using natural or organic soil, occasional supplementation might be necessary depending on your soil's baseline or water quality. However, it's advisable to start feeding at a lower strength and increase gradually. Over-fertilizing can lead to nutrient burn—a common mistake that slows growth and damages the plant's delicate leaves.

Many growers follow a feeding schedule tailored specifically to the vegetative phase, adjusting nutrient concentrations as the plants grow larger and their needs increase. A light feeding during early veg with a gentle formula followed by a ramp-up to a fuller nutrient program feels natural and supports steady development without overwhelming the plants. If you're new to feeding, consider using pre-formulated nutrient mixes designed for cannabis veg stages to simplify this part of the process.

Beyond the type and amount of nutrients, how you deliver them matters. The watering routine often doubles as your feeding schedule—watering with nutrient-enriched water so roots receive consistent access to essential elements. Yet, it's important not to feed fertilized water every time you water; alternating with plain pH-balanced water can flush excess salts and minerals, preventing buildup in the soil.

Remember, cannabis plants are sensitive to changes, especially during the vegetative phase when they're rapidly building biomass. Sudden shifts in light hours, watering habits, or nutrient levels can cause stress, slowing growth or causing leaf deformities. Keeping a steady, predictable routine helps your plants settle into a healthy growth pattern and maximize their vegetative potential.

Growing cannabis is as much about observation as it is about schedules and measurements. Learn to read your plant's leaves and overall posture. Dark green, sturdy leaves without spots indicate healthy nitrogen levels and proper light exposure. Yellowing edges or curled tips might hint at nutrient imbalances or watering stress.

Early detection lets you adjust before major problems arise, helping maintain a smooth vegetative phase that sets your crop up for larger yields down the line.

Overall, this stage is your chance to build a plant's strength and size. Smart management of light cycles, precise watering, and thoughtful nutrient feeding create the foundation for a bountiful harvest. Don't rush, don't overdo it, and don't underfeed your enthusiasm. Take time to dial in each factor carefully—consistent routines and patient attention pay dividends when you move on to flowering and bud development.

Plant Training Techniques for Bigger Yields

Once your cannabis plants reach the vegetative stage, it's the perfect time to start training them. Training shapes your plants, improves light penetration, and ultimately helps you harvest bigger, denser buds. Whether you're growing a single plant or managing a small garden, mastering plant training techniques during this early stage can make a huge difference in how well your crop performs down the line.

At its core, plant training is about controlling how your cannabis stretches and fills out. Instead of letting the plant grow naturally in a tall, skinny shape with one main cola, training encourages bushier, more even growth. This means more flowering sites and better exposure to light for all parts of the plant. When done right, this not only increases yield but can also improve airflow, reducing the risk of mold and pests later during flowering.

There are two broad categories of training: low-stress training (LST) and high-stress training (HST). Low-stress training focuses on gently bending and repositioning branches to control growth without causing damage or shock. High-stress techniques, on the other hand, involve pruning, topping, or other more aggressive methods that cause intentional trauma, spurring the plant to grow stronger and bushier as it heals. Both categories have their place, and many growers combine them for maximum effectiveness.

One of the most popular low-stress training methods is simply bending and tying down branches. As your plant grows, you gently pull the tips outward and downward, securing them with soft ties or garden wire to the sides of your container or grow tray. This flattens out the canopy, creating what's often called a "manifold" or "screen of green" shape. You'll notice that instead of one dominant top cola, you get multiple smaller tops all growing evenly, which means a bigger surface area for developing buds. It's a gentle way to encourage growth without stressing a young plant.

Another simple LST technique involves using a trellis net or screen above your canopy. As branches grow through the net, you tuck and weave them back under, creating a more uniform horizontal plane. This method is especially helpful if you're growing multiple plants close together because it helps maximize the use of your grow space. Plus, it forces lower bud sites to receive more light, improving their quality.

High-stress training techniques include topping, fimming, and supercropping. Topping involves cutting off the main shoot just above a node, where two new branches will then grow, essentially doubling the number of colas. This encourages a wider, bushier plant. Fimming is similar but less precise—you pinch off part of the growing tip instead of cutting it cleanly. Both methods work by redirecting the plant's energy from upward growth to lateral branches.

Supercropping is a more advanced HST technique where you intentionally "bruise" the inner tissues of a branch by gently bending it until it softens but doesn't break. This signals the plant to divert extra nutrients and hormones to that area, strengthening the branch and promoting more vigorous growth. Though it sounds intimidating, with practice, supercropping can greatly enhance your plant's structural integrity and yield potential.

Choosing which training methods to use depends on your grow space, the strain you're cultivating, and your personal preferences. Indicas typically respond better to topping since they're naturally shorter and bushier, while sativas, which grow taller and stretch more, might benefit more from LST and supercropping to control height. A hybrid strain might require a mix of both approaches.

Timing is key with all these techniques. The vegetative stage is the best window because your plants are still flexible and resilient enough to handle stress without slowing down their growth. Start training once the plants have at least three to five nodes and always monitor their response closely. Pushing too hard or too early can stunt development, while waiting too long could result in missed opportunities for canopy control.

Another important consideration is the plant's overall health during training. Nutrient levels, watering, and light intensity all play a role in how well your plants recover from manipulation. A stressed plant won't react well to topping or bending, so keep your environment optimized and consistent. Healthy foliage and strong stems make the process smoother and your results more predictable.

Don't underestimate the value of patience and observation. Every plant reacts differently—even within the same strain and grow setup. Take notes on how each individual responds to training, and adjust your approach accordingly. Being attentive helps you fine-tune techniques for bigger, better yields while minimizing setbacks.

Training isn't just about maximizing your yield — it's also a form of plant management that keeps growth under control, especially in limited spaces. Indoor growers often face height restrictions, so bending and topping help prevent plants from hitting grow lights or tents. Outdoor growers, meanwhile, use training to protect plants from wind damage and to expose more bud sites to the sun's rays.

As you progress through vegetative growth, keep up with trimming and pruning as needed. Remove smaller, shaded branches that won't develop into quality buds. This conserves the plant's energy and enhances airflow, which helps prevent mold and pest issues later in the cycle.

Ultimately, the goal is to create a balanced, even canopy that makes the most of your light and space. Well-trained plants produce more uniform buds that mature evenly, making harvest day more rewarding and efficient. With consistent training during the vegetative stage, you're setting the stage for bountiful, high-quality yields.

Don't be discouraged if your first attempts at training seem awkward or slow. It's a skill that improves with time, observation, and a bit of trial and error. The investment is well worth it, as these techniques unlock the true potential of your cannabis plants and bring your growing skills to the next level. Remember, successful cultivating combines patience, attention to detail, and a willingness to adapt your methods according to what your plants need.

Spotting Healthy Growth in Vegetative Stage

When you reach the vegetative stage in your cannabis grow, it's like the plant is hitting the gym and bulking up. This is the time when the plant focuses on building strong stems, lush foliage, and a solid root system to support future flowering and bud development. Knowing what healthy growth looks like during this phase is vital to catching any issues early and making adjustments that will lead to a thriving harvest.

First off, color is one of the simplest indicators of health. Well-nourished cannabis leaves during the vegetative stage will have a vibrant, rich green tone. Light or yellowing leaves often signal nutrient imbalances, particularly nitrogen deficiencies, which are almost always a concern during this rapid growth phase. On the flip side, very dark green leaves could hint at nutrient burn, so keep an eye out for any signs of discoloration that stray from that healthy medium green.

A healthy plant's leaves should look full and robust, not fragile or droopy. Sufficient turgor pressure, which is the strength from water inside the cells, helps leaves stand upright and firm. Wilting or curling could mean anything from under- or overwatering to heat stress or even root problems. When you inspect your plants, note how the leaves react — are they perky and waving towards the light, or are they hanging limply?

Another aspect to monitor is new growth. Healthy cannabis plants won't just maintain their current leaves; they'll be producing fresh shoots regularly. You want to see symmetrical growth patterns with evenly spaced nodes (the points on a stem where leaves develop), signaling that the plant is distributing its energy well and growing with balance. If new leaves seem unusually small, malformed, or stunted, it may point to stress factors like improper lighting, pH imbalance, or nutrient deficiencies.

Stems and branches also give clues about plant vigor. Strong, thickening stems support the weight of the canopy as it expands throughout this stage. If stems feel thin or brittle, or if you notice drooping branches, your plant might be struggling to transport water and nutrients properly. Give your plants enough space to stretch and develop sturdy branches, and this will pay off during flowering when heavy buds need solid support.

Root health ties directly into what you see above the soil. While you can't see roots without disturbing the plant, the overall vigor of the plant often reflects the condition underground. Healthy roots are white and fibrous, full of root hairs, and spread comfortably within the growing medium. If you suspect issues—such as slow growth or yellowing leaves—check the roots carefully. Dark, slimy, or foul-smelling roots are signs of root rot and need immediate attention.

Environmental factors also influence how healthy your vegetative plants look. Temperature, humidity, light intensity, and airflow will all impact growth rates and leaf condition. Cannabis thrives in moderately warm temperatures (65°F to 80°F) during the day with slightly cooler nights. Excessive heat will make leaves curl and dry out, while cold can slow growth and cause discoloration.

Humidity levels should remain balanced as well. High humidity risks mold and mildew, whereas too dry conditions can cause leaf tips to crisp and yellow. The correct humidity for vegetative growth usually falls between 40% and 70%, depending on your setup. Maintaining fresh air circulation reduces stagnant conditions that encourage pests and diseases, promoting healthier leaves and stems.

When you're monitoring vegetative growth, pay close attention to how your plants respond after watering and feeding. Healthy cannabis will absorb water well without showing immediate signs of stress such as wilting or leaf curling. Overwatering often causes yellow leaves to appear at the bottom since roots can't breathe properly. Underwatering leads to droopy leaves that don't bounce back quickly. Developing a keen eye for these differences helps you keep your watering routine on point.

One more thing to look for is the plant's overall shape and structure during this stage. Ideally, your plants should exhibit a strong, balanced canopy with plenty of lateral branching alongside the central stem. This formation indicates a good genetic foundation and proper care. Plants that stretch excessively (get "leggy") may need a little more light, while those that grow short and tight might be a sign that light intensity or quality is sufficient, or possibly that genetics are playing a role.

Another subtle but important indicator involves leaf edges and tips. Under ideal conditions, leaf edges should be smooth and tips intact. If you observe browning or curling at the tips or edges, this might point to minor nutrient burn, pH swings, or a slight temperature spike. These issues are often fixable before becoming serious problems, so consistent observation will give you the chance to intervene early.

Remember, growth isn't always perfectly linear. Plants often fluctuate with environmental changes and feeding schedules. What really matters is the overall trend—steady improvements in leaf size, color, and stem strength over days and weeks. If you notice emerging signs of stress, act promptly by adjusting your grow environment, feeding, or watering rather than waiting for deterioration.

It helps to develop a routine where you visually inspect each plant daily during the vegetative stage. Use this time to not only check for healthy growth but also spot early signs of pests like spider mites, aphids, or fungus gnats that can quickly affect the plant's development. Keeping a grow journal or log can steadily improve your ability to detect patterns and troubleshoot effectively as you gain experience.

Overall, spotting healthy growth in the vegetative stage blends observation, attentiveness, and a little bit of intuition. Knowing what a thriving cannabis plant looks like provides a solid foundation for the next stages, ensuring your efforts pay off with vigorous flowering and bountiful yields. This stage is your chance to lay down the roots—literally and figuratively—for a successful cannabis journey ahead.

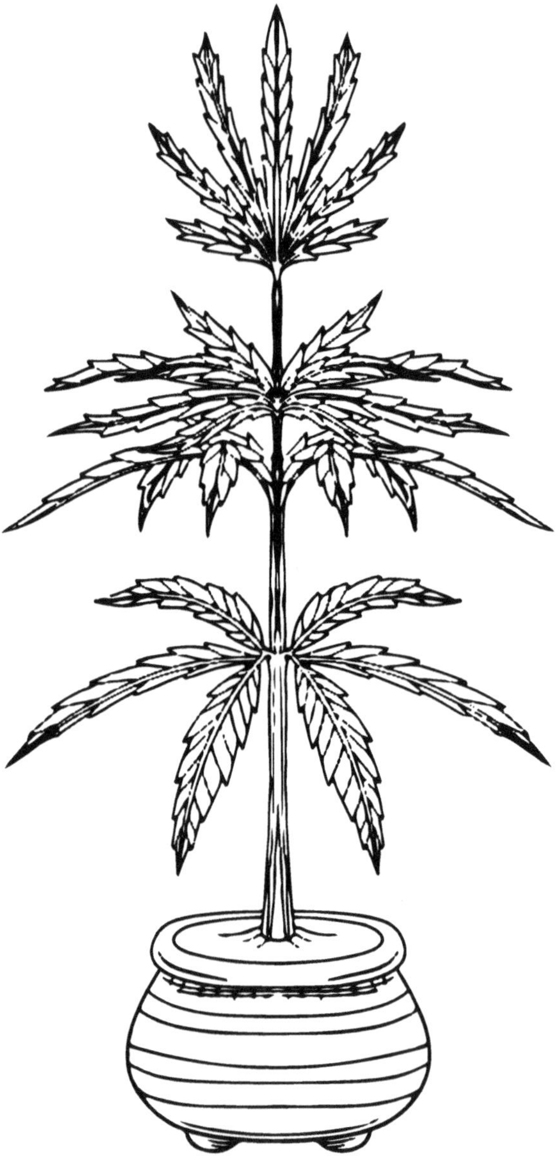

Chapter 6
The Flowering Stage

This phase marks the exciting transition where your cannabis plant shifts focus from growing leaves and stems to producing buds, the ultimate goal of any grower aiming for a quality harvest. Triggered by changes in light cycles—typically reducing light exposure to 12 hours a day indoors—the flowering stage demands careful attention as your plants develop rich, resinous flowers that signal nearing maturity. During this time, managing environmental factors like humidity and airflow becomes crucial to prevent mold and ensure bud density, while controlling the plant's smell may require odor management solutions in indoor grows. Success in flowering means closely watching your plants' progression, adjusting nutrients accordingly, and preparing for the rewarding task of harvest by recognizing the subtle visual cues that hint when your buds are reaching peak potency. Staying engaged every step of the way maximizes your crop's flavor, aroma, and overall quality, transforming weeks of work into a thriving, fragrant reward.

Triggering Flowering for Indoor Cultivation

Transitioning your cannabis plants from the vegetative phase into flowering is a critical step in indoor cultivation. Unlike outdoor grows—where seasonal changes naturally cue this shift—indoor environments give you full control over the process. Mastering how and when to trigger flowering lets you optimize bud quality, manage your grow space efficiently, and ultimately set the stage for a successful harvest. Since lighting schedules are the primary trigger for flowering indoors, this section will dive into practical strategies that help you confidently make that switch.

At its core, initiating flowering indoors means altering your light cycle to mimic the natural progression from summer into fall. Cannabis is a photoperiod plant, which means it reacts to the amount of daily light it receives. During the vegetative stage, plants thrive on long hours of light—typically 18 to 24 hours per day. When you reduce light exposure to about 12 hours, you simulate shorter days, signaling your plants to shift energy from growing leaves and stems to developing flowers. This change is essential; if the light cycle isn't adjusted properly, your plants may remain stuck in vegetative mode or develop unevenly.

The most common light schedule used to trigger flowering indoors is the 12/12 cycle—12 hours of uninterrupted darkness followed by 12 hours of light. It might sound simple, but each aspect of this schedule demands careful attention. Uninterrupted darkness is crucial; even small light leaks during the dark period can confuse plants and lead to problems like hermaphroditism or stalled flowering. Many growers go to great lengths to create a completely light-tight growing space—using blackout curtains, sealing gaps, or even lining grow tents with reflective but opaque materials to ensure consistent darkness.

Keep in mind that timing matters just as much as duration. Ideally, you set a consistent "lights off" and "lights on" time every day. Plants adjust their internal rhythms based on this predictability, which helps promote healthy flowering. Flickering lights or irregular schedules can stress plants, reducing yield and quality. Using timers is a must for indoor growers; modern digital timers offer the precision and reliability necessary to maintain strict cycling without manual errors. Once you switch to the flowering light cycle, be prepared to follow it daily until harvest without interruption.

Beyond simply switching the light schedule, consider how your lighting setup impacts the flowering phase. The type of lights you use can influence the speed and quality of bud development. During flowering, many growers prefer high-intensity light sources with a spectrum rich in red wavelengths, as red light encourages flowering and bud formation. High Pressure Sodium (HPS) and certain full-spectrum LEDs are popular choices. While you don't need to overhaul your lighting entirely, adjusting your light spectrum or swapping bulbs can push your plants toward healthier, denser flowers.

When it comes to the actual process of triggering flowering, many cultivators wait until their plants reach a certain size or maturity before flipping the light cycle. Generally, plants should be strong and healthy with a solid vegetative structure that can support substantial bud growth. Switching too early—when plants are small or underdeveloped—can stunt overall yield. Conversely, waiting too long means longer total grow times and potentially larger plants that may crowd your space. Monitoring plant size, node count, and overall vigor will guide your decision on when to initiate flowering indoors.

It's also worth noting that some growers choose to train their plants during the vegetative stage to maximize flowering potential once the light schedule changes. Techniques like topping, low stress training (LST), or screen of green (ScrOG) can create an even canopy, increasing light penetration during flowering. While training itself doesn't trigger flowering, it prepares plants so the transition is more productive. The combination of well-timed flowering triggers and strategic plant management sets the stage for bigger, more uniform buds.

Understanding your cannabis strain's genetics is another crucial factor when triggering flowering. Indica, sativa, and hybrid strains each respond differently to the shift in photoperiod. Indicas typically flower faster and may require shorter vegetative periods, while sativas often benefit from longer vegetative growth before flowering. Some strains are known to be more sensitive to light interruptions or inconsistent schedules. Familiarizing yourself with your seeds' flowering preferences helps you tailor your lighting strategy, avoiding common pitfalls like delayed flowering or hermaphroditism.

When flipping to a flowering schedule, keep environmental conditions stable. Temperature, humidity, and airflow should all be adjusted to support flowering plants, which generally require slightly cooler temperatures than during vegetative growth. However, sudden environmental changes can stress your plants during this sensitive period. Maintain moderate temperatures around 65 to 80 degrees Fahrenheit and keep humidity lower—around 40% to 50%—to reduce risks of mold and mildew in your dense buds.

Don't overlook the importance of regular monitoring during this stage. After triggering flowering, keep a close eye on your plants for signs of stress, light burn, or nutrient deficiencies. Sometimes, plants react strongly to the change in light cycle, exhibiting yellowing leaves or slowed growth, which signals that adjustments might be needed in feeding, watering, or environmental controls. Remember, flowering demands more energy and resources from your plants—nutrient needs will shift too, but feeding details come later.

Some growers experiment with "sexing" plants during early flowering once you've triggered the process. Identifying male plants early is essential to prevent pollination and seed production, which detract from bud quality. While the exact timing varies by strain, flowering is when pre-flowers and pistils become visible, allowing you to separate males swiftly. Triggering flowering is not just about inducing buds, but also about managing your crop to target only female plants for optimal harvest.

While fluorescent and LED lights are common in the vegetative stage, flowering typically calls for bulbs that provide more intense and specific light spectrums, as mentioned. Additionally, inspecting your grow space for light leaks is an ongoing task. Even if you think your room is sealed, small gaps behind vents or cables entering the tent can introduce stray light. Inconsistent dark cycles are one of the easiest ways to throw off flowering, resulting in stretched buds, lower potency, or hermaphroditic plants. There's no shortcut here—successful flowering demands disciplined control of your light environment.

Beyond light and environment, your flowering trigger also marks a mental shift in how you manage your grow. Plants become more sensitive to overwatering or nutrient imbalances, so it's essential to adjust your care routine with the increased demands of flowering. This phase is the payoff for all your earlier efforts, so giving flowering plants what they need in terms of light, space, and environment will maximize your harvest's size and quality.

Finally, patience is vital here. Flowering times vary by strain, generally lasting between 6 and 12 weeks after triggering. Don't rush the process by interrupting or modifying your light schedule once you've switched. The buds need consistent signals to mature fully. If you maintain a steady 12/12 cycle and stable environmental conditions, you'll help your plants produce the dense, resinous flowers that make all the effort worthwhile. By mastering how to trigger flowering indoors, you take one of the most critical steps toward successful, rewarding cannabis cultivation.

Bud Development and Maturity Indicators

As your cannabis plants transition fully into the flowering stage, the excitement builds with the appearance of buds, those dense, resinous flowers that hold the sought-after cannabinoids and terpenes. Understanding how buds develop and knowing when they reach maturity is crucial for every grower looking to maximize quality and potency. Bud development isn't just a visual milestone—it's an intricate biological process influenced by genetics, environment, and nutrient availability. Recognizing key maturity indicators helps you decide the optimal harvest time, ensuring your efforts pay off with top-shelf cannabis.

Bud growth starts at the calyxes, tiny teardrop-shaped structures that multiply and cluster on the plant's flowering nodes. Early in the flowering phase, these calyxes are small and tightly stacked, almost fragile to the touch. As flowering progresses, they swell, gaining weight and depth, gradually transforming into larger, more robust buds. The pistils—hair-like structures emerging from the calyxes—begin white and wispy but turn darker and curl inward as the buds age. Tracking this pistil color transition is a common method used to estimate maturity, though it should be combined with other indicators to avoid premature or late harvests.

One of the most reliable maturity indicators lies in the tiny glandular trichomes peppered over the buds, sugar leaves, and even stems. These trichomes produce the resin that contains cannabinoids, terpenes, and flavonoids, giving cannabis its distinctive effects and aroma. Watching trichome development requires a magnification tool, like a jeweler's loupe or handheld microscope. As buds mature, trichomes shift from clear and translucent to a milky white or cloudy appearance. This change signals peak cannabinoid production and potency. Eventually, trichomes turn amber-colored, indicating cannabinoid degradation and a shift towards a more sedative effect. Deciding when to harvest often boils down to the right balance of milky and amber trichomes, depending on your desired effects.

Aside from trichomes and pistils, other subtle signs hint at bud readiness. The overall bud density increases dramatically; mature buds feel firm and sticky, a sign that resin has fully developed. The aroma intensifies, filling the grow space with a pungent, complex fragrance unique to each strain. You might also notice the surrounding sugar leaves curling slightly or fading in color as the plant reallocates energy to the buds. On the plant level, fan leaves might yellow and die back near harvest time, a natural indicator that the plant is winding down its lifecycle.

Environmental stress during flowering can influence bud development, sometimes speeding up or stalling maturity. Temperature swings, light intensity changes, and nutrient imbalances all play a role. For instance, insufficient phosphorus or potassium during flowering can stunt bud swelling, leaving you with airy, underdeveloped flowers. Consistent monitoring and adjustment throughout flowering help maintain healthy bud growth. Equally important is managing humidity levels to prevent mold or mildew in dense buds, ensuring your crop remains clean until harvest.

Patience during bud development pays dividends. Many growers fall into the trap of harvesting too early, attracted by the sight of mature-looking pistils but missing crucial resin development within trichomes. Early harvests often result in less potent, harsher smoke that lacks the full flavor profile of a fully mature bud. Conversely, waiting too long risks cannabinoid degradation and an overly sedative or "couch-lock" effect that may not suit everyone's preferences.

Besides the technical indicators, getting familiar with your strain's typical flowering period sets realistic expectations for bud maturity. Some indica-dominant strains finish faster, with dense, chunky buds reaching maturity in as few as seven weeks of flowering. Sativa-dominant strains usually take longer, often ten weeks or more, producing looser, fluffier buds with slower resin development. Hybrids fall somewhere in between, depending on their genetic makeup. Tracking your plants' progress week by week and noting changes helps build your experience bank, letting you tailor your harvest decisions more confidently in future grows.

From a practical standpoint, documenting bud development with photos throughout flowering creates a valuable reference. Visual records help you recognize the subtle differences between early, peak, and late flowering stages on your specific strains. This habit also sharpens your ability to read trichomes and pistils accurately, especially when paired with magnification tools. Over time, you'll develop an intuitive sense for the optimal harvest window, boosting your success rate consistently.

In addition to internal maturity cues, ready buds respond to gentle touch differently. Immature buds feel spongy and pliable, while mature ones resist compression, springing back slightly. Sticky resin coats the buds and sugar leaves, making handling noticeably tacky. Experienced growers often use these tactile cues alongside visual ones for a more rounded assessment. Yet, it's always best to rely primarily on trichome inspection, as this provides the most direct insight into cannabinoid development.

During late flowering, pay attention to how buds fill out their spaces on the plant. Ideally, clusters should be compact and exhibit fully formed pistils and a heavy trichome covering. Buds typically grow larger and tighter around the main colas (the top bud sites on branches) but keep an eye on lower buds, too. Smaller "popcorn" buds rarely reach the same quality or density, so many growers opt to prune and focus energy on main flower sites earlier in the grow.

Remember that bud maturity isn't just about size—it's about chemical composition. A bud that looks massive but hasn't developed white, milky trichomes probably isn't ready. Conversely, a smaller, denser bud with ample mature trichomes may be far beyond the earliest signs of quality. This distinction matters both for effect and consumer satisfaction, whether you're growing for personal use or to share with others.

Overall, mastering bud development and maturity means paying close attention to evolving pistil colors, trichome shifts, bud density, aroma, and tactile feel. Each factor provides clues, but together they form a complete picture of readiness that no single sign can fully express alone. Your role as a grower is to observe, learn, and adjust your timing for the unique behavior of your plants, creating an ideal balance between waiting long enough for optimal potency and harvesting before degradation begins.

In the end, successful flowering hinges on understanding these development stages and maturity indicators well. It's a rewarding phase in your grow cycle where patience, observation, and knowledge combine to produce the buds you've worked so hard to cultivate. With practice, you'll gain the confidence to make timely harvest decisions that elevate your cannabis to its fullest potential, whether you seek a euphoric cerebral high, deep relaxation, or full-spectrum medicinal benefits.

Managing Smell and Space During Flowering

The flowering stage is where all the hard work you've put into your cannabis plants really pays off. However, it's also when managing the physical space and controlling the intense aromas becomes crucial. As buds develop and mature, the smell of your grow room can become very potent—something to prepare for early on, especially if discretion is a priority. At the same time, the plants will expand and fill out, requiring smart spatial planning to avoid overcrowding and ensure each bud gets enough light and airflow.

First off, let's talk about the smell. Cannabis buds are known for their strong, distinctive odor during flowering because of the increased production of terpenes, which are the compounds responsible for scent and flavor. This aromatic punch can be a double-edged sword—it's exactly what gives your harvest its character, but it also makes keeping your grow discreet a bit trickier. Luckily, there are practical solutions to keep the smell in check while letting your plants flourish.

One of the most effective ways to manage odors is by investing in a quality carbon filter attached to your ventilation system. Activated carbon filters are specifically designed to trap and neutralize odors before the air leaves your grow tent or room. Coupled with a powerful exhaust fan, this setup can significantly reduce the scent escaping into your living space or outdoors. It's worth noting that, for best results, the air filtration system should be running constantly throughout the flowering period; turning it off, even temporarily, risks releasing a strong aroma that neighbors or visitors might notice.

Besides carbon filters, some growers use additional odor-neutralizing products that work in conjunction with air exchange systems. These can include ozone generators, specialized odor-absorbing gels, or natural solutions like activated charcoal bags placed strategically nearby. Keep in mind, though, that ozone generators require careful handling because excessive ozone can harm both your plants and your health. Choose products carefully and consider safer, passive methods before resorting to more aggressive techniques.

Another tip is to keep your grow room or tent sealed as well as possible. Check for air leaks around openings, seams, and doors. Even small gaps can let odors escape and reduce the efficiency of your filtration system. Seal any gaps with weather stripping or tape designed for grow environments. This not only helps with smell control but also with maintaining consistent temperature and humidity, both of which are vital during flowering.

Now, regarding space—flowering plants can get surprisingly bushy. You might have started with a neat, manageable setup in the vegetative stage, but as flowers swell, branches can crowd each other. This crowding reduces light penetration and airflow, which can lead to problems like mold and mildew. Managing space effectively means planning for your plants' maximum size and training them during earlier stages to optimize canopy shape. If you end up with a dense mass of foliage, bud development suffers, and so does overall yield quality.

One straightforward method to manage space is to use plant training throughout flowering, but since training techniques are covered elsewhere, let's focus here on spatial arrangements and environmental adjustments. Giving each plant ample room in your grow tent or room promotes healthy airflow around buds, which helps reduce the risk of wet spots where mold can take hold.

Remember, stagnant air combined with dense flowers is a recipe for disaster, especially in humid climates.

For indoor growers constrained by limited space, consider staggering the height of your plants or using scrog (screen of green) nets to spread out canopy evenly. These strategies help fit more bud sites within the same square footage without the plants shading one another excessively. A well-managed horizontal spread also makes maintaining and harvesting easier, since you can get good access to every bud without damaging other parts of the plant.

Another aspect to keep in mind is vertical space. Flowering cannabis can grow surprisingly tall even after switching photoperiods, especially with some sativa-dominant strains. This growth can quickly surpass the height limits of grow tents or rooms. Anticipate this by either choosing strains known for moderate height or by cropping and topping plants early enough to control vertical stretch. If your space is small, using low-stress training (LST) before flowering can prevent dramatic stretching, letting you maximize yield while still fitting comfortably within your setup.

It's also smart to monitor your grow environment's temperature and humidity closely as plants bloom and bulk up. The extra biomass increases transpiration rates, meaning your HVAC setup might need adjustment to keep conditions ideal. Proper humidity control is key to preventing mold growth, particularly in tight quarters where airflow might be limited by the sheer number of flowers. Dehumidifiers and oscillating fans can be essential tools here, especially when combined with open, uncluttered spacing.

At times, it's tempting to cram in as many plants as possible, especially during your first few grows. However, overcrowding backfires by creating stress and increasing disease risk, which results in fewer, lower-quality buds. Fewer well-spaced plants will almost always outperform overcrowded batches in potency, aroma, and overall health. Patience and planning here can make a huge difference.

Don't overlook the importance of regular maintenance and cleaning during flowering. Remove dead leaves and debris routinely so they don't accumulate and contribute to odors or pest problems. Some growers segment their flowering area and go through a daily or every-other-day clean-up routine to keep things under control. This ongoing attention helps maintain optimal airflow and prevents hotspots for smells or pathogens.

Lastly, if odor is still a major concern due to neighbors, family, or legal restrictions, look into blower silencers and ducting methods that further channel and minimize sound and scent escaping. Soundproofing your grow area can also help avoid drawing unwanted attention during the flowering period. Remember that the goal is to keep your grow as discreet and pleasant as possible while nurturing your plants to full maturity.

To sum up, managing smell and space during flowering requires a balance of good equipment, thoughtful plant care, and strategic environmental control. Using carbon filters, sealing your grow space, spacing plants for airflow, and monitoring humidity keeps your grow healthy — and your odor contained. Meanwhile, planning for vertical and horizontal growth avoids overcrowding and stress. If you take these steps seriously, you'll create the perfect atmosphere for your buds to develop dense, flavorful flowers without headaches or surprises along the way.

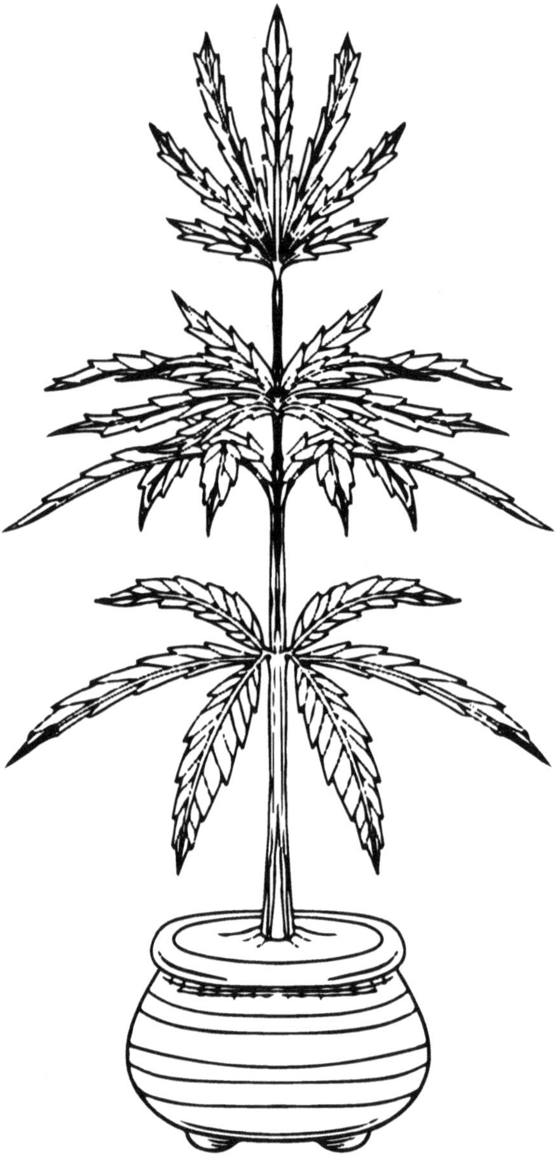

Chapter 7
Harvesting Like a Pro

Knowing when and how to harvest your cannabis plants can truly make or break your final product, so this stage deserves your full attention and care. It's about more than just cutting down buds—it's recognizing the subtle signs that signal peak potency, like the color shifts in trichomes and pistils, which tell you the exact moment to reap the rewards of your hard work. Using the right tools and techniques prevents damage and preserves the precious cannabinoids and terpenes, ensuring your buds retain flavor, aroma, and strength. With a solid plan in place, harvest day transforms from a nerve-wracking task into a satisfying culmination of weeks of dedication, priming you for the next phases of drying and curing that lock in quality.

When to Harvest: Reading Trichomes and Pistils

Knowing precisely when to harvest your cannabis plants can make a significant difference in the quality and potency of your final product. This timing often hinges on two key indicators on the plants themselves: trichomes and pistils. Becoming adept at reading these markers is essential for anyone looking to elevate their growing game from average to pro level. While it's easy to feel overwhelmed at first, especially if you're new to cultivation, understanding these signs will empower you to harvest at the perfect moment every time.

Trichomes are the tiny, resinous glands that coat your cannabis buds and leaves. They look like minuscule crystals or frosted sugar dust when viewed with the naked eye and appear as tiny mushroom-shaped structures under magnification. These glands are where cannabinoids like THC and CBD, as well as terpenes responsible for aroma and flavor, are produced and stored. As your plant ripens, trichomes change in both appearance and potency, making them a reliable indicator of maturity.

To properly inspect trichomes, a good magnification tool is crucial. Many growers use a jeweler's loupe with 30x to 60x zoom or a digital microscope that connects to a smartphone. By closely examining the color and clarity of trichomes, you can determine the ideal harvest window for your specific strain and desired effects.

Initially, trichomes appear clear, indicating they are still immature and haven't reached their peak cannabinoid levels. At this stage, harvesting would result in a less potent and less flavorful product. As the plant matures, trichomes turn milky white or cloudy and then eventually shift to an amber hue. The cloudy stage typically signals the peak THC content, offering the highest psychoactive potential. When a portion of the trichomes starts to amber, some of the THC begins to degrade into CBN, a cannabinoid that produces more sedating effects. So, if you want a more energetic, euphoric high, aim to harvest when most trichomes are cloudy. But if you prefer a calming, couch-lock vibe, waiting until some trichomes have turned amber may be better.

Keep in mind, not all trichomes on a single plant will transition at the exact same rate. It's normal to see a mix of clear, cloudy, and amber trichomes on different buds or parts of the plant. Your goal is to find a balance that matches the effect profile you're targeting. Also, environmental factors like temperature and humidity can influence these changes, so closely monitoring your grow conditions can help you predict the right harvest time.

Pistils—the fine, hair-like structures that emerge from the calyxes of female cannabis plants—offer another vital clue about harvest readiness. Early in the flowering phase, pistils tend to be long, thin, and white, standing straight out from the buds. As the plant matures, these pistils darken and curl, changing from white to shades of orange, red, or brown. Watching this color transformation is a classic, easy-to-see method for growers to estimate when the buds are nearing maturity.

However, pistil color alone doesn't tell the full story. Some growers harvest too early just because 50% or more of the pistils have darkened, but trichomes tell a fuller story about cannabinoid development. Pistils can sometimes change color before the trichomes reach their peak potency. That said, pistils provide a solid initial gauge and are especially useful when you don't have access to magnification tools.

Most cultivators wait until roughly 70% to 90% of the pistils have darkened and curled before considering harvest. If you harvest too soon, when most pistils are still white, the buds might not have fully developed THC and flavor profiles. On the flip side, letting all pistils darken and curl can mean the plant has passed its prime, leading to a more sedative effect and slightly reduced potency. It's a balancing act, and observing pistils alongside trichomes provides the clearest picture.

It's worth noting that different strains can show variability in trichome and pistil development. Indicas usually mature faster than sativas and might have pistils that darken more quickly. Hybrids may show a blend of these timelines. Your familiarity with your chosen strain's typical flowering times will help you interpret these signs better and avoid premature or delayed harvests.

Environmental stress can also influence trichome and pistil appearance, so it's important to maintain stable conditions during flowering. Sudden temperature shifts or fluctuations in humidity can cause trichomes to degrade prematurely or pistils to change color erratically, leading to confusing harvest signals. Keeping a consistent grow environment reduces these risks and helps ensure your trichomes and pistils develop naturally and predictably.

As you approach the end of the flowering stage, make it a habit to check your plants daily or every other day using a magnifier. This frequency helps catch the subtle changes, so you don't miss the perfect harvest window. Harvesting just a few days too early or late can shift the flavor and effect profile drastically. Patience and attention to detail at this point pay off with a more potent and flavorful yield.

Another tip is to pick a couple of representative buds from different areas of your plant for close inspection. Often, buds nearer the top may mature faster due to better light exposure, while lower or shaded buds take longer. Sampling multiple spots ensures you're harvesting when the majority of your crop is ready rather than just a few select colas.

In some cases, growers prefer to fine-tune harvest timing based on the intended use of their harvest. For medicinal users prioritizing relaxation, waiting longer for amber trichomes might maximize sedative cannabinoids. Recreational users seeking an uplifting experience might harvest earlier when trichomes are mostly cloudy. Experimenting with these harvest windows over successive grows is a great way to dial in perfect timing for your personal goals.

It's helpful to record your observations about trichome and pistil development in a grow journal. Tracking dates alongside photos and color notes helps you better predict timing for future grows of the same strain. Over time, this documentation becomes an invaluable resource that elevates your cultivation skills and confidence.

When it's finally time to harvest, remember that this decision should weigh heavily on the combined evidence from reading both trichomes and pistils. Relying on just one can lead to less-than-ideal results. Together, these indicators create a fuller story about your plants' readiness and help you capture the quality and potency every grower aims for.

To summarize, mastering the art of reading trichomes and pistils takes some practice but delivers significant rewards. By observing trichome color shifts—from clear to milky to amber—and monitoring pistil darkening and curling, you gain a solid, practical method for timing your harvest. The right timing amplifies the cannabinoid concentration, terpene expression, and overall experience your buds provide. For cannabis enthusiasts and growers who want to cultivate with precision and maximize their crop's potential, these natural signs are your most trustworthy guides.

Tools Essential for a Successful Harvest

When it comes to harvesting cannabis like a pro, having the right tools at your fingertips can make all the difference between a smooth, efficient process and a frustrating, damaging ordeal. You want to be prepared to handle every step carefully—from cutting down your plants to trimming the buds with precision. Using the right equipment not only helps maintain the quality of your harvest but also reduces the risk of contamination, wasted product, and unnecessary wear on your plants.

One of the most fundamental tools you'll need is a reliable pair of trimming scissors or shears. These aren't just any scissors; they should be sharp, sturdy, and specifically designed for trimming cannabis. Good trimming scissors make it easier to work quickly and neatly, ensuring you don't crush delicate buds or lose precious resin glands. Many growers prefer ergonomic designs that reduce hand fatigue since trimming can be a time-consuming task. It's worth investing in a quality pair that's comfortable to hold and sharp enough to glide through stems and leaves cleanly.

Alongside scissors, you'll also want to have a sharp, durable knife on hand. A well-maintained pruning knife or a straight-edged razor blade is invaluable for making the initial harvest cut on your plants. These tools help you swiftly cut the main stalk or branches without crushing or tearing. Keep in mind that hygiene is paramount;

sterilizing knives and scissors before use helps prevent infections or mold issues later during drying and curing.

Another tool that might not seem obvious but proves indispensable is a magnifying glass or a jeweler's loupe. While this is often used before harvest to inspect trichomes, it's also helpful right at harvest time to double-check buds or spot small leaves that need trimming. A loupe with at least 30x magnification gives you a clear view of trichome clarity, which is crucial to harvest timing—but that's something we cover in another section. For now, just remember that having a loupe on hand means you can maintain quality control right through the cutting and trimming process.

Harvesting can create quite a mess, so it's a good idea to have clean surfaces and containers ready for collecting your trimmed buds. Many growers use trays or mats specifically made for trimming cannabis. These surfaces keep your workspace tidy and prevent tiny trichomes and sticky resin from being lost. Non-stick trimming mats also make cleanup easier and can help preserve the delicate aromas and valuable trichomes that you don't want to waste.

Gloves are another essential tool that's sometimes overlooked. Wearing disposable nitrile gloves helps keep your hands clean and prevents oils, dirt, and sweat from transferring onto your buds. Plus, gloves protect you from the sticky resin, which can be tough to wash off and clog your trimming scissors over time. Using gloves also helps minimize your scent footprint on the harvest, allowing you to keep the aroma fresh and uncontaminated.

Of course, as your harvest volume increases, you might consider specialized trimming machines. While hand trimming is usually superior for preserving bud quality, these machines can help save time if you're dealing with a large crop. Trimming machines use rotating blades and catch trays to remove leaves quickly. However, they require practice to avoid damaging buds and removing too many trichomes. Many pros choose to do a rough trim with machines followed by a careful hand trim to ensure the best results. Trimming machinery comes in varied sizes, so select one that matches your grow operation's scale.

Storage containers play a role immediately after harvest. Airtight jars or food-grade containers help keep trimmed buds safe while they await drying and curing. It's best to have several sizes on hand—from small containers for delicate, high-value nugs to larger ones for bulk storage. Glass jars with sealing lids work well because they don't impart odors or chemicals into the buds. Avoid plastic bags because they can crush the flowers and degrade quality. Labeling containers by strain and harvest date can be incredibly useful when managing multiple crops or experimentation batches.

In addition to harvesting and trimming tools, you'll want some measuring and monitoring gear nearby. A small digital scale can help you track your yields with accuracy. This is especially helpful if you're focused on improving your cultivation skills and want to compare results across different grows. Keeping records of weight at harvest can also motivate you and guide your adjustments in the next grow cycle. While not strictly necessary, a scale is a practical investment for any serious grower.

Light is another consideration during harvest. Though you don't need intense grow lights at this stage, having a well-lit workspace is crucial. Good lighting allows you to spot fine details when trimming and reduces mistakes. Portable LED lights or adjustable desk lamps are a fantastic option. They help you keep an eye on trichomes, pistils, and the overall health of your buds while working. Also, bright but cool lighting won't cause heat stress or degrade your crop as you handle it.

Keeping your tools clean throughout the harvest process is vital. Cannabis resin can build up quickly on blades and scissors, dulling their effectiveness and spreading contamination. You should have cleaning supplies like isopropyl alcohol and soft cloths ready to regularly wipe down your equipment. Cleaning your tools after significant trimming intervals maintains sharpness and prevents resin from gumming up the works. The cleaner your tools, the smoother your trim and the better the final quality.

Sometimes you might also want to include harvest-specific accessories such as buckets or garbage bins lines with compostable bags. These containers make it easier to dispose of fan leaves and excess plant material without cluttering your work area. Keeping your harvesting zone tidy reduces the risk of mold and helps keep pests away from freshly cut buds. Consider designating an area just for waste that's separate from your trimmed flower to stay organized during the busy harvest period.

Harvesting cannabis requires patience and precision, and that mindset goes hand in hand with having the right gear. As your skills grow, you'll develop your preferred toolkit, but these basics will get you through a professional-quality harvest. Investing in quality tools not only speeds up the entire process but also preserves the integrity of your crop, boosting both potency and flavor. After all, a remarkable harvest starts well before cutting—it begins with being ready and equipped to do the job right.

Finally, don't forget that comfort matters. Harvesting can take hours, sometimes days, depending on the size of your grow. Wearing comfortable clothing, having enough seating or padding for your knees, and making sure your workspace is ergonomic can make this labor-intensive phase more enjoyable. When you feel good physically, you work better, trimming more carefully and appreciating the fruits of your labor.

With the right set of essential tools, you'll be equipped to tackle your harvest confidently and efficiently. These items form the backbone of every grower's success and help transform the final stage of cultivation into a rewarding experience instead of a stressful chore. Harvest time truly is the moment when all your efforts bloom into reality, so making it as smooth as possible with the proper tools will ensure every nug shines as brightly as it can.

Step-By-Step Harvesting Checklist

Harvesting cannabis is the critical moment where all your hard work finally comes to fruition. Knowing exactly what to do, and when, will help you preserve the plant's potency, flavor, and overall quality. To confidently bring your crop from growth to usable product, it pays to follow a clear, detailed checklist. Whether this is your first harvest or your tenth, sticking to a reliable plan will minimize mistakes and maximize yield.

Start by preparing your harvest workspace in advance. Cleanliness is essential. Clear away clutter, sanitize your tools, and set up a well-lit area with plenty of ventilation. Having everything within reach will keep the process smooth—you don't want to fumble looking for scissors or gloves once you begin cutting. Spread out clean trays or parchment paper to lay out branches as you trim to avoid contamination.

Next, gather the right tools. Sharp, sterile pruning shears or scissors are a must to make clean cuts and prevent damage or unnecessary stress to the buds. Rubber gloves can help protect your plants from oils on your skin and keep your hands sticky-free. You might also want magnifying glasses or a jeweler's loupe handy to inspect trichomes up close, ensuring you harvest at peak potency.

Timing is everything. Before diving into cutting, double-check your plants' maturity. Look for primarily milky white or cloudy trichomes with some amber ones mixed in, signifying optimal THC levels and flavor. Also, inspect the pistils—the hairs on buds—making sure most have darkened and curled away from the flower. Rushing the harvest too early or waiting too long will affect the final product's effects and taste.

Now, begin the actual harvest by cutting whole branches or individual cola tops, depending on your drying space and method. For indoor grows, trimming branch by branch allows better airflow during drying. Outside, you might opt to harvest entire plants at once if space permits. Be gentle with your cuts to avoid knocking off precious trichomes, which hold much of the plant's cannabinoids and terpenes.

Once branches are severed, it's time to remove large fan leaves. These don't contain as much resin and only add extra moisture and weight. Pull or cut them off carefully, but don't stress the buds. Some growers perform a "wet trim" at this stage, trimming smaller sugar leaves right away; others wait until after drying. The right choice depends on your setup and preference, but consistency in your approach pays off.

Place freshly cut and trimmed branches on drying racks or hang them upside down in a dark, cool, well-ventilated space. Ideal drying conditions are around 60-70°F with 50-60% humidity. Good airflow helps prevent mold and preserves aroma. Drying typically takes 7 to 14 days; buds should feel dry on the outside but still slightly spongy inside. If they crumble too easily, they risk losing potency.

While buds dry, inspect for any signs of mold or pests daily. If you spot suspicious spots or unusual smells, address the problem immediately by improving airflow or adjusting humidity. Prevention here is better than curing, as once mold sets in, your harvest can be ruined. Patience during drying is key—don't rush this step, as it directly impacts smoothness and flavor when smoking or vaping.

After buds reach the right dryness, it's time for the final trim—removing any remaining small sugar leaves and manicuring the buds into an appealing shape. This not only improves appearance but also helps with curing, allowing the buds to breathe and release moisture evenly. Save trimmed leaves and small buds for concentrates or edibles instead of discarding them.

Once manicured, transfer the buds to airtight containers for curing—usually glass jars work best. Open the jars daily for the first couple of weeks to "burp" the buds, letting excess moisture escape while fresh air takes its place. This gradual process enhances flavor and potency by allowing biochemical changes within the cured cannabis. Keep jars in a cool, dark place for at least 2-4 weeks, though longer curing yields even better results.

Throughout harvesting, keeping detailed notes is often overlooked but incredibly valuable. Record the harvest date, harvest conditions, drying times, and any observations on the smell or appearance of the crop at each step. This info will help you refine techniques for your next grow and troubleshoot potential issues before they escalate. A grow journal can become a grower's best friend over time.

Another tip worth mentioning: make sure to stay hydrated and take breaks. Harvesting can be surprisingly labor-intensive—both mentally and physically. Keeping your workspace organized and your mind sharp avoids mistakes like accidentally cutting too much or missing signs of ripeness. Approach each stage with care and focus; treating your plants respectfully during harvest honors the effort you put into growing.

Remember, the hoopla around harvest day can tempt you to rush, but cannabis cultivation rewards patience and precision. Following this checklist not only safeguards your yield's quality but also enhances its final effects and enjoyment. Over time, the steps of harvesting will become as natural a part of your routine as watering or pruning.

By mastering this step-by-step harvesting checklist, you're completing a vital chapter in your cannabis growing journey. Each phase—from workspace prep to jar burping—is crucial to turning fresh plants into premium buds. Stick with the process, learn from each cycle, and watch how your harvests improve season by season.

Chapter 8
Drying and Curing Essentials

Once you've harvested your cannabis, the drying and curing stages are crucial to transforming those freshly cut buds into a smooth, potent, and flavorful product. Drying properly means controlling the environment—temperature, humidity, and airflow—for several days to a couple of weeks until the buds feel dry but not brittle. This step slows down chlorophyll breakdown and prevents mold, which can ruin your crop. After drying, curing takes this process further by storing your buds in airtight containers that are periodically opened to release moisture and gases, allowing the flavors and potency to develop fully over weeks or even months. Skipping or rushing these steps can lead to harsh smoke, diminished effects, or even mold issues. Paying close attention during drying and curing will reward you with cannabis that tastes better, burns evenly, and delivers the quality you worked so hard to achieve.

How to Properly Dry Cannabis Buds

Drying cannabis buds is a crucial step in the journey from harvest to a perfectly cured product. You've put in months of hard work growing, nurturing, and harvesting your plants. Now, if the drying process isn't handled correctly, all that effort can be undermined by poor flavor, mold, or harsh smoke. Drying isn't just about removing moisture; it's about preserving cannabinoids, terpenes, and the overall integrity of your buds. Get this right, and you'll set yourself up for a rewarding curing phase that can bring out the best characteristics of your cannabis.

First things first, timing and environment are the foundation of proper drying. The goal is to slowly remove moisture from the buds without causing them to dry too fast or stay wet too long, which can create mold issues. Typically, a steady drying period lasts about 7 to 14 days, but this can vary depending on environmental conditions and the size of the buds. What you're aiming for is a slow, controlled process—one that gradually brings the moisture level down to around 10-15%. This balance is key for flavor preservation and smooth smoke.

Humidity control plays a starring role here. Ideally, you want relative humidity in your drying space to hover around 45-55%. Too dry, and the buds can become brittle, leading to loss of terpenes and a harsh experience. Too humid, and mold becomes a real threat. Temperature is equally important, with an ideal range sitting between 60-70°F (15-21°C). Staying within these parameters helps encourage the slow breakdown of chlorophyll, which reduces the grassy, hay-like taste often associated with rushed drying.

How you hang your buds matters, too. Most growers opt to hang whole branches or trimmed buds upside down in a clean, dark room with good airflow. Hanging allows air to circulate freely around each bud, helping to avoid moisture pockets that can foster mold. When hanging branches, be sure there's enough spacing between them—crowding can trap moisture and slow drying. If space is tight, trimming buds before drying on drying racks is also a solid alternative.

Regarding airflow, it needs to be gentle and consistent. A small oscillating fan helps keep air moving but don't point it directly at your buds. Direct airflow can dry the outer parts of the buds too quickly, sealing in moisture deeper inside, which can lead to mold after the drying phase. A balanced breeze ensures moisture evaporates evenly without stressing the plant material.

Light exposure is another factor to control. Exposure to light, particularly UV rays, can degrade cannabinoids and terpenes. Maintaining total darkness in the drying area is often recommended. Darkness protects the precious compounds while also reducing chances for heat buildup in the drying space. This is something attention-worthy, especially when drying cannabis in warmer climates or with suboptimal room setups.

Now, how do you know when your buds are properly dried? A simple test is to gently squeeze a bud between your fingers. It should feel dry on the outside but slightly spongy and not brittle. The small stems attached to the buds should snap rather than bend. If the stems still feel flexible, your buds need more drying time. On the other hand, if the buds crumble or snap too easily, they are likely over-dried.

During the drying process, keep an eye out for any signs of mold or mildew. If you spot white fuzzy spots or a musty smell, act immediately. Remove any infected buds to prevent contamination of the entire batch. Also, check the drying environment's humidity and airflow, adjusting as needed to stop further mold growth. Being proactive here can save a harvest from total loss.

One practical tip is to monitor the drying progress daily. Opening the drying space to check humidity levels, air circulation, and bud condition is crucial. Many growers use hygrometers to track the environment's humidity and temperature continuously. This data helps fine-tune conditions early and often, avoiding the common pitfalls of drying too quickly or too slowly.

Patience is a virtue during this stage. The temptation might be to rush things to get to the curing phase, but slow and steady drying pays off in richer flavor profiles and smoother smoke. Rushed drying often results in harsh buds that burn hot and taste grassy or chlorophyll-heavy. Remember, drying sets the tone for the entire post-harvest quality. If done right, it maximizes the potential locked in those trichomes.

Many experienced growers recommend drying in a closed, dedicated room or closet to keep environmental factors consistent. This space should be clean, free of dust and pests, and equipped with a small heater or dehumidifier if needed to control humidity. If you're drying in a humid climate, a dehumidifier can be a lifesaver, preventing the stubborn mold problems that plague many outdoor and basement drying setups.

Freshly harvested cannabis might still have a significant amount of water inside the buds and branches, so don't expect the drying process to finish quickly. Often, environmental variables like altitude and season will impact drying rate. Cooler temperatures usually slow drying, while warmer temperatures speed it up but increase risk of terpene loss. Adjust your approach accordingly: sometimes ambient conditions demand a little creativity, like running a low-temperature fan or opening a window during drier parts of the day.

Another important aspect involves pretreatment before hanging. Some growers prefer "sweating" freshly cut branches for 12-24 hours in large paper bags or cardboard boxes to begin moisture equalization before actual drying. This can gently kick off moisture release without shocking the buds into drying too fast. However, care must be taken to avoid creating a humid environment that encourages mold growth. This method isn't necessary for everyone but can be an interesting approach to experiment with if you're aiming for an artisanal product.

While drying is mostly about reducing water content, it's also the phase when fragile trichomes, those tiny resin glands rich in cannabinoids and terpenes, can deteriorate if handled improperly. Avoid rough handling of buds during drying. Using gentle hands when trimming or handling dried branches helps keep these glands intact, preserving potency and aroma. Some growers even dry buds on mesh racks to avoid direct contact and minimize damage.

Lastly, know that drying is a prelude to curing—not the end itself. Proper drying prepares your buds for curing by stabilizing moisture content. Once drying is complete, your buds will be fragile but not brittle, and this is the perfect moment to transition into controlled curing environments. Patience again plays a central role; rushing from harvest straight to consumption without this step risks losing a significant part of your crop's quality and potential.

The entire drying phase educates you on your cannabis's true character and teaches respect for the plant's delicate nature. With focus on humidity, temperature, airflow, and handling, you're protecting what makes cannabis special—the flavors, the aromas, and the unique effects. Whether you grow just a few plants for personal enjoyment or launch into larger batches, mastering proper drying sets you apart as a conscientious cultivator. And with every successful dry, you move closer to that perfectly cured, premium-quality cannabis you worked so hard to produce.

Curing Techniques for Maximum Potency and Flavor

Once you've successfully dried your cannabis buds, the next crucial step is curing. This often-overlooked process can make a dramatic difference in the potency, flavor, and overall quality of your final product. Curing is essentially an art form combined with a science, involving carefully controlled storage conditions that allow the cannabis to mature beyond drying. During curing, biochemical reactions break down unwanted byproducts and enhance cannabinoids and terpenes, the compounds responsible for potency and aroma.

The goal here is to slowly remove residual moisture from the buds while preserving the delicate trichomes that house the active compounds. If you rush curing or skip it, you could end up with harsh smoke, muted flavor profiles, or even diminished effects. In contrast, a well-cured stash offers a smoother, more potent experience with rich, nuanced flavors that deepen over time. For growers aiming to elevate their crop from just good to exceptional, mastering curing is essential.

Begin curing by placing your thoroughly dried cannabis buds into airtight containers, typically glass jars.

Glass is preferred due to its non-reactive properties and ability to maintain stable humidity. Avoid plastic, as it can impart off-flavors and doesn't offer the same humidity control. Fill the jars about 75% full to allow some airflow inside without squishing the buds. Overpacking the jars can create excess moisture pockets that risk mold development.

Proper humidity control during curing is critical. Ideal relative humidity (RH) for curing sits in the 58-65% range. Maintaining this range prevents buds from drying out too quickly or getting too moist, both of which can degrade quality. If the buds are too dry going in, they won't cure properly and can become brittle. Too much moisture, on the other hand, invites mold, mildew, and poor flavor. Small humidity packs made specifically for cannabis curing are a convenient way to regulate RH inside your jars, ensuring consistent conditions without daily monitoring.

After sealing your jars, the curing process requires daily "burping" for the first one to two weeks. Burping means opening the jars briefly—about 10-15 minutes—to let fresh air circulate and release any built-up moisture. This exchange prevents stale air and excess humidity from accumulating. Pay close attention during this period; if condensation appears on the inside of the jar, that signals too much moisture, and you may need to leave the jar open a little longer or remove some wetter buds. After the initial phase, you can reduce burping frequency to a few times per week.

Temperature also impacts curing outcomes. Maintaining a cool environment around 60-70°F (15-21°C) is optimal for preserving cannabinoids and terpenes. High temperatures accelerate terpene evaporation and cannabinoids' breakdown, which reduces aroma and potency. A dedicated curing space free from direct sunlight and temperature swings helps keep the buds stable. Avoid places prone to fluctuations, such as near vents or windows, which can stress your crop during this delicate phase.

The entire curing process can last from two weeks up to three months, depending on your goals. Many growers find a good balance at around four to six weeks, where buds have mellowed significantly and exhibit a rich flavor profile. Extending curing beyond two months can sometimes improve flavors further but demands vigilant moisture control to prevent degradation or mold. Experienced cultivators often taste test periodically, using their nose and smoothness of the smoke as a guide to decide when the curing has peaked.

One interesting aspect of curing is its effect on potency. While some cannabinoids might degrade slightly during curing, the overall effect often feels stronger. This happens because harsh chlorophyll and other undesirable chloroplast compounds break down, making the experience smoother and more enjoyable.

Terpenes, responsible for distinctive cannabis aromas, develop more fully and change subtly with curing, unveiling hidden bouquet notes that were previously masked. Essentially, curing lets the plant's full character emerge, which can transform how you appreciate your homegrown harvest.

It's worth mentioning that curing conditions may vary slightly for different strains. For example, dense indica buds might need more vigilant burping early on, since denser flowers trap moisture more than airy sativa buds. Hybrid strains often fall somewhere in between. Understanding how your particular genetics respond to curing can refine your technique over multiple grows. Keep notes on humidity, temperature, and burping schedules to develop a customized approach that consistently yields superior results.

Advanced growers sometimes experiment with curing variations, such as "in-jar" curing contrasted with traditional hang-and-dry followed by jar storage. Some even try curing with oxygen absorbers or controlled nitrogen environments to preserve freshness for longer. While these methods can push quality further, they require precise monitoring tools and experience. For most home cultivators, simple jar curing with controlled humidity and frequent burping strikes the right balance between ease and great results.

Another tip to maximize curing success is to handle buds gently during the process. Excessive handling can knock off fragile trichomes, reducing potency and diminishing appearance. Resist the urge to constantly open the jars just to inspect. Instead, trust your drying stage to get you close to the right moisture level, and let curing do its slow work without too much disturbance.

In addition to jars, some growers use specialized containers like humidity-controlled curing boxes or vacuum-sealed bags post-initial cure phase. These options can protect your cured cannabis longer but might not offer the same nuance of control. Whether you opt for basic glass jars or invest in specialized equipment, consistency is key. A steady curing environment will reward your patience with buds that smoke perfectly and showcase the best your grow had to offer.

Finally, be cautious of common curing mistakes: storing freshly harvested buds without drying, neglecting to burp jars, or storing at excessively high temperatures. Each of these errors can quickly lead to mold, off flavors, or loss of potency. By following a disciplined curing routine, you enhance cannabinoid preservation and terpene retention, producing a more enjoyable and powerful final product.

In short, curing is where your cannabis transitions from a raw harvest into a refined, premium product. It's a step that requires patience, attention to detail, and the right environment but pays off handsomely by unlocking flavors and effects you won't get otherwise. Whether you're aiming to impress friends or simply want the most satisfying smoke for yourself, understanding and mastering curing techniques is an indispensable skill for elevating your homegrown cannabis to its fullest potential.

Avoiding Mold and Rot During Post-Harvest

After the excitement of harvest, the attention to detail during the drying and curing phase becomes critical in preserving the quality of your cannabis. One of the biggest challenges growers face right after harvest is avoiding mold and rot. These issues not only destroy the potency of your buds but can also ruin entire batches if left unchecked. Mold and rot thrive when moisture lingers too long in the buds, so controlling the environment and handling your cannabis carefully are key to preventing these problems.

First off, timing plays a huge role. Hanging your branches or placing trimmed buds in a drying space that's too humid or poorly ventilated creates the perfect storm for mold spores to take hold. Ideally, you'll want to dry your cannabis in a well-ventilated area with temperatures ranging from 60 to 70 degrees Fahrenheit and relative humidity between 45 to 55 percent. These conditions help moisture evaporate steadily, reducing the chances that damp spots develop inside dense buds where mold loves to grow.

One mistake many growers make is rushing the drying process or leaving buds to dry in an overcrowded space. When buds are packed too tightly or hung too close together, airflow becomes limited. This trapped moisture, especially in the inner layers of the flower, invites botrytis cinerea, commonly called bud rot, and other molds. Spread your branches out evenly or use mesh racks with enough space between buds to encourage consistent airflow around every piece. Using fans strategically can help circulate air, but avoid blowing wind directly on drying cannabis, as this can cause uneven drying and degrade trichomes.

Another important step is trimming your buds properly before or after drying. Many growers trim after drying because it helps buds lose moisture more evenly. Removing excess leaves and stems reduces the overall moisture content that hangs around, which also lowers the risk of mold forming. That said, some cultivators prefer a wet trim, where they cut leaves before drying but must be extra vigilant about maintaining ideal drying conditions. Whichever method you choose, make sure buds aren't sitting in clumps or sealed containers until they're dry enough.

Monitoring your drying space regularly will save you headaches later on. Check your humidity and temperature with reliable meters and adjust as needed. If humidity spikes, dehumidifiers can bring levels back down quickly. Conversely, adding moisture with a small humidifier or simply leaving a shallow tray of water nearby can raise humidity if it gets too dry, which can crack and dry buds too fast, leading to harsh smoke. Avoid rapid drying; too much heat or dryness can degrade cannabinoids and terpenes, and it makes buds more brittle and less flavorful.

Once drying is complete, curing provides another layer of protection against mold and rot, but it's not immune to problems either. Improper curing—such as sealing buds in airtight containers that aren't monitored—creates pockets where moisture can build up again. As buds continue to slowly breathe out moisture during the first weeks of curing, you'll need to burp your jars or containers daily to release excess humidity. This process keeps the internal environment stable and prevents condensation, which could lead to mold growth.

Containers used for curing should be clean, dry, and ideally made from glass or food-safe materials that don't trap odors or off-gas chemicals. Plastic bags and certain plastics can promote sweating or create uneven humidity. Glass mason jars with airtight seals are a classic choice, offering good protection while allowing easy monitoring. If you notice any musty or sour smells, inspect your buds carefully for early signs of mold. Moldy buds should be removed immediately to avoid contamination spreading.

Handling your harvested cannabis with clean, dry hands or gloves also helps avoid introducing mold spores. Dirty tools, surfaces, or hands can transfer unwanted microbes onto your precious buds. Sterilizing scissors, trimming trays, and drying racks between uses is a small step that makes a big difference. In addition, ensure your drying and curing area is free from dust, pet hair, and other contaminants that could settle on your buds.

Keep in mind that genetics and plant health before harvest impact how susceptible your buds are to post-harvest mold and rot. Plants stressed by pests, nutrient imbalances, or environmental factors tend to produce denser buds that retain moisture more stubbornly, so managing plant health throughout the grow cycle helps enormously. However, even top-notch genetics and perfect cultivation can be undone by careless post-harvest handling.

Investing in a hygrometer or humidity controller that logs data over time can give you peace of mind by tracking environmental changes during drying and curing. Some growers opt for small packs designed to regulate humidity inside curing jars, such as Boveda packs, which maintain a steady 62 percent humidity level ideal for curing cannabis buds. These can reduce the need for frequent burping and add an extra layer of protection against mold development.

It's also wise to set up your drying area in a space that's separate from your grow area to avoid cross-contamination. Mold spores can travel through the air easily, so having a clean, dedicated spot for drying and curing reduces your chances of accidental infections. Maintaining good airflow, avoiding stagnant pockets, and keeping temperatures steady all work together to keep your buds healthy through these delicate final stages.

In summary, the key to avoiding mold and rot during post-harvest lies in controlling moisture and airflow, paying close attention to environmental conditions, and handling buds with care. Slow and steady drying, combined with careful curing practices, preserves the essential cannabinoids and terpenes that make your cannabis enjoyable and potent. Your efforts here will pay off with clean, flavorful, mold-free buds that enhance your overall cultivation success.

CHAPTER 9
STORAGE AND PRESERVATION METHODS

Once your cannabis is perfectly dried and cured, storing it correctly becomes crucial to maintaining its potency, aroma, and overall quality over time. The key is to protect your buds from light, heat, air, and moisture, all of which can degrade cannabinoids and terpenes if not managed well. Using airtight containers in a cool, dark place helps slow down deterioration, while avoiding plastic bags or containers that can trap humidity or generate static. Proper storage isn't just about keeping your stash fresh; it's about preserving the experience you worked hard to cultivate, so you can enjoy those rich flavors and effects whenever you want. Taking a few extra steps now ensures your harvest stays effective and enjoyable long after the growing season ends.

Best Practices for Long-Term Cannabis Storage

Preserving your cannabis for the long haul is an essential skill every grower needs to master, especially if you're aiming to keep your buds fresh, potent, and flavorful over months or even years. It's more than just tucking your harvest into a dark corner and hoping for the best. Proper long-term storage means controlling factors that can break down cannabinoids and terpenes or invite mold, degradation, and loss of aroma. Whether you're saving a personal stash or storing a big harvest, knowing the right techniques can make a world of difference in how your cannabis ages and performs.

First off, understanding what damages cannabis over time is crucial. Light, heat, air, and moisture are the primary enemies when it comes to preserving potency and quality. Exposure to even low levels of light speeds up degradation of THC and other cannabinoids, making your buds less effective. High temperatures accelerate chemical changes and can also encourage mold growth if combined with humidity. Oxygen—while necessary for life—oxidizes cannabinoids, turning that freshly-harvested peak into a dull, dry product. Lastly, improper humidity levels either dry out buds to the point of crumbling or trap moisture that fosters mold development.

So, how do you fight all these factors? The answer lies in creating a stable microenvironment tailored specifically for cannabis. Using airtight containers is your first line of defense. Mason jars, especially those made of glass, are the go-to choice since they don't impart flavors and seal tightly to limit airflow. Plastic bags or containers, on the other hand, can leach chemicals and often aren't airtight enough. For long-term storage, aim for containers that you can open a few times without weakening the seal. Avoid squeezing or compacting your buds too much as that can damage the trichomes—those tiny resin glands packed with cannabinoids and terpenes.

Temperature control can't be overstated. Ideally, cannabis should be stored in a cool place, generally between 60°F and 70°F. Sudden temperature fluctuations damage cannabinoids and terpenes as they expand and contract, breaking down the chemical structure and aroma profile. Refrigerators might seem like a good option, but they can create moisture issues and promote mold if the humidity isn't balanced correctly. Avoid freezing your buds as well; freezing damages the trichomes and often results in a crumbly texture once thawed.

Humidity is another aspect that warrants close attention. Maintaining relative humidity (RH) between 55% and 62% helps preserve the moisture content of buds without promoting mold. Too dry, and your cannabis will lose its sticky texture and flavorful profile, turning brittle and harsh. Too moist invites mold and can render your harvest unsafe to use. To manage humidity accurately over long periods, many growers add humidity control packets—these nifty little sachets are calibrated to maintain ideal RH inside sealed containers. By incorporating them, you keep your stash consistently fresh without worrying about frequent monitoring.

Light exposure is a silent assassin of cannabis quality. Ultraviolet (UV) rays from sunlight degrade THC and other cannabinoids, so keep your storage containers in a dark place. Opt for opaque storage boxes, or if you're using clear jars, stash them inside a cabinet or drawer away from any direct or ambient light. Many growers personalize this with a dedicated stash box lined with blackout materials or place their jars inside a closed cupboard specifically reserved for cannabis storage. The goal is to minimize any chance for light to sneak in.

Of course, long-term storage practices don't stop at simple containment. It's just as important to consider how you manage your stash on a day-to-day basis. Resist the temptation to open your containers repeatedly, which introduces fresh oxygen and moisture fluctuations. Organize your storage so you're grabbing your cannabis from one sealed jar at a time rather than constantly cycling air in and out. This reduces the risk of degradation drastically. Some growers even label jars with packaging dates and strain types, making rotation easier and helping them use the oldest product first.

When it comes to the actual preparation of cannabis before storage, trimming and curing play a role. Overly wet or inadequately cured buds won't store well since residual moisture invites mold. Make sure your buds are dried and cured properly to lock in flavors and reduce moisture content. If you store cannabis too wet or too dry, you'll face problems over time. Proper curing also protects cannabinoids against oxidation by encouraging slow chemical stabilization during the curing period. But once curing is complete, storing your buds in airtight containers under the right conditions will maintain that quality.

One consideration experienced growers often mention is the benefit of vacuum sealing. Removing air from your storage container can significantly slow oxidation, but vacuum sealing carries risks if not done properly. Excessive compression can crush trichomes, and without controlling humidity inside the bag, your flowers may dry out completely. Employ vacuum seal only when you have a reliable way to maintain the ideal humidity level inside the package, or use it in combination with humidity control packs. It's also best used for shorter-term storage since prolonged lack of airflow can lead to other issues.

Another effective method is using airtight silicone containers, which are great for maintaining trichome integrity when dealing with concentrates or cannabis flower. Silicone isn't porous and can withstand temperature swings better than plastics or glass, reducing the risk of mold. Some growers prefer this method for small quantities they plan to consume quickly, but it can be a part of your strategy depending on the size of your stash and frequency of use.

Let's not forget that every cannabis strain is unique, and while core storage principles remain the same, certain strains with higher terpene content may be more sensitive to storage conditions. Terpenes are what give cannabis its distinctive aroma and play a role in the overall experience. Preserving these aromatic oils requires even more care with temperature, light, and humidity. For premium strains or those you want to savor at their absolute best, investing in high-quality storage containers with better seals and temperature control features will pay off.

Aside from the physical factors, hygiene plays a subtle but vital role in long-term storage success. Before packing your buds, clean your jars or containers thoroughly to prevent contamination. Dust, residual moisture, or leftover particles can introduce mold spores or bacteria that flourish in sealed environments. Use warm water and mild detergent, then dry completely to avoid trapping moisture inside. If you're storing cannabis for very long periods, consider cleaning your storage space regularly and monitoring conditions—dust buildup or pest activity can spoil your efforts.

When storing cannabis for long-term, it also makes sense to avoid storing multiple strains in the same container. Each strain carries a distinct terpene profile that can blend or clash when mixed, diluting the unique flavors and aromas you worked hard to develop. Separate storage helps keep your collection organized and ensures each bud retains its identity. It's a small detail but important for curators and collectors who treat cannabis like a craft product rather than just a commodity.

As your stash grows and ages, regular checks can help catch early warning signs of trouble. Periodically inspect your storage jars for signs of mold, bud dryness, or any odd smells. Catching problems early prevents potential ruin. If you spot mold, discard the affected buds immediately and sanitize your storage area. Smells can also change due to terpene degradation or contamination; fresh cannabis has a vibrant, characteristic aroma, while stale or poorly stored material tends to turn musty or flat. Trust your senses as part of your long-term storage routine.

Lastly, consider how you plan to consume your cannabis when choosing long-term storage methods. If you're preserving flower for smoking, maintaining that sticky, resinous quality is critical. For those interested in medicinal use, it might be more important to preserve potency and cannabinoid profiles. For making extracts later, the preservation of terpenes still matters but often takes a backseat to cannabinoid preservation. Tailoring your storage approach to your end use will help you get the most value from your harvest through time.

In summary, long-term cannabis storage demands intentional control over environment, container choice, and handling. Stay consistent about keeping your buds cool, dark, airtight, and properly humidified. Avoid rapid temperature changes, excessive air exposure, and repeated container opening. Cleanliness and organization support the quality preservation process while strain separation and regular inspection protect your investment. Watching how your cannabis ages builds invaluable knowledge, helping you refine your approach on future grows and keep every harvest as potent and fresh as the day you brought it in.

How to Maintain Potency and Freshness

Once you've put in the hard work of growing, harvesting, drying, and curing your cannabis, maintaining its potency and freshness becomes just as crucial as the cultivation process itself. Proper storage is the bridge that preserves all your efforts, ensuring that your buds deliver the experience and effects you expect, long after harvest season. Without careful attention to storage conditions, cannabinoids like THC and terpenes degrade over time, causing your once-potent stash to lose its potency, aroma, and overall quality.

The first rule of maintaining potency and freshness is managing your cannabis' exposure to the elements.

Cannabis is sensitive to oxygen, light, heat, and humidity, and each can have detrimental effects on potency. Oxygen initiates the degradation process that breaks down THC into CBN, which is far less psychoactive. Light, especially UV rays, can degrade cannabinoids and terpenes, diminishing both the strength and flavor of your buds. Heat can accelerate chemical breakdown and cause trichomes, the resin glands packed with cannabinoids and terpenes, to become brittle and fall off. Humidity, if not controlled properly, can promote mold growth or cause the buds to dry out and lose their sticky, resinous quality.

One of the best ways to maintain freshness is to store cannabis in airtight containers that limit oxygen exposure. Glass jars with tight-sealing lids remain the go-to choice for most growers. Avoid plastic bags or containers that aren't airtight — these allow oxygen to seep in and hasten degradation. Mason jars are affordable, reusable, and generally easy to find. Opt for smaller jars if you're storing limited quantities to avoid repeatedly exposing your entire stash to air during each use. This not only conserves potency but also retains the full flavor profile over time.

Temperature control plays a major role. Cannabis should ideally be stored at a cool, stable temperature, often considered around 60-70°F (15-21°C). Storing in warmer environments invites terpene evaporation and cannabinoid degradation. Additionally, frequent temperature swings can cause moisture buildup or drying, both detrimental to quality. Avoid places like kitchens, windowsills, or near heating appliances. Instead, opt for a dark cupboard, closet, or even a dedicated humidity-controlled cannabis storage box.

Humidity is just as important as temperature. Aim to keep relative humidity (RH) between 55% and 62% for optimal cannabis preservation. Too much moisture can lead to mold and mildew growth, problems that ruin entire batches and pose health risks. On the flip side, extremely low humidity dries buds out excessively, causing harsh smoke and loss of terpenes. Many growers use humidity packs designed to maintain stable RH levels inside storage containers. These handy packs balance moisture without letting the buds become damp or brittle, preserving their texture, look, and potency.

Light exposure must be limited entirely since it triggers cannabinoid breakdown. Always keep your cannabis in a dark environment. Glass jars are great, but if they're clear, consider wrapping them in cloth or storing in a box to shield from light. Avoid plastic containers that let light through easily, as this can significantly reduce potency over a relatively short period. When cannabis is stored in amber or dark-colored glass jars, this can also help block out harmful UV rays and prolong freshness.

Another often-overlooked factor is minimizing handling. Every time you open your storage container, you introduce fresh oxygen and humidity fluctuations that accelerate degradation. It's a good idea to store smaller quantities separately, so you only open what you plan to use immediately. Using clean, dry tools to handle your cannabis keeps contamination and unwanted moisture to a minimum. Be mindful that frequent, careless handling can also cause existing trichomes to break off, reducing the overall cannabinoid content.

For those looking to preserve cannabis for the long haul — months or even years — consider vacuum sealing as an option. Vacuum sealing removes excess oxygen from the packaging, significantly slowing the oxidation process. While this method is popular in commercial settings, home growers should only vacuum seal properly dried and cured cannabis to avoid trapping moisture inside, which can lead to mold. It also helps to store vacuum-sealed bags in cool, dark places to optimize preservation. Be aware that over time, the vacuum seal can weaken, so periodic checks are wise.

Freezing is another method sometimes used for long-term storage, yet it comes with precautions. If you're planning to freeze cannabis, the buds must be fully cured and dried to prevent ice crystals from forming inside trichomes, which can cause them to rupture. Store in an airtight container with added humidity control and place in the freezer quickly to reduce moisture exposure. When opening frozen cannabis, allow it to come to room temperature in its sealed container before breaking the seal to avoid condensation forming on the buds. Despite these precautions, freezing is less common among home growers due to the risk of trichome damage and is generally better suited for concentrates.

Proper labeling and organization also contribute indirectly to maintaining potency and freshness. Keeping track of harvest dates, strains, and storage conditions allows you to rotate stock wisely, using older buds first and avoiding lengthy storage of material beyond its prime window. Some strains preserve better than others, so monitoring your stash encourages better decision-making for future harvests and storage methods.

In summary, the keys to holding onto your cannabis' potency and freshness revolve around limiting oxygen exposure with airtight containers, controlling temperature and humidity, protecting buds from light, and minimizing frequent handling. By understanding how cannabinoids and terpenes react to environmental factors, you can create an ideal haven that keeps your harvest as vibrant and flavorful as the day you harvested it. Thoughtful storage goes beyond just putting buds in a jar—it's a continuous process that pays dividends in the quality and experience of your cannabis.

Remember, investing effort into maintaining freshness will reward you with enhanced effects, richer aromas, and a more satisfying experience. Whether you're a beginner or a seasoned grower, these storage strategies form an essential part of your cultivation blueprint that ensures your crop's full potential is unlocked every time you reach for it.

Avoiding Contamination in Stored Cannabis

Proper storage of cannabis is about more than just keeping your buds fresh—it's a critical step in preserving their quality and safety. One of the most overlooked aspects of storage is preventing contamination, which can easily ruin your harvest and pose health risks. Whether you're storing small amounts for personal use or planning for long-term preservation, avoiding contaminants like mold, bacteria, and unwanted pests should always be a top priority.

The first line of defense starts with cleanliness. When cannabis is stored, any dirt, dust, or foreign particles present in the container or environment can transfer to the buds. Those particles might harbor bacteria or mold spores ready to colonize under the right conditions. It's essential, therefore, to use storage containers that are clean and preferably sterilized. Glass jars with airtight seals remain the gold standard because they don't absorb odors or moisture and are easy to sanitize. Avoid plastic bags or containers since they can trap moisture and degrade over time, creating a perfect breeding ground for contaminants.

Another common source of contamination often comes from handling. Every touch introduces new microbes, oils, and even dirt from your hands to the flowers. Always wash your hands thoroughly before handling your cannabis or use clean gloves to minimize contamination. This is especially important if you're transferring buds between containers or inspecting them during curing or storage. A simple preventative habit like this can drastically reduce the risk of unwanted mold and bacterial growth.

Environmental factors also play a huge role in contamination risks. Cannabis stored in humid or poorly ventilated spaces can quickly develop mold, especially if excess moisture is present. Moisture levels above 62% relative humidity are generally risky for mold growth, while anything below 55% can cause the buds to dry out and lose potency. Using humidity-control packets like Boveda or Integra Boost can help maintain a sweet spot, preventing both mold and overly dry cannabis. These packets are designed to keep your cannabis at optimal moisture levels without the guesswork.

Temperature control is equally important. Storing cannabis in warm environments accelerates degradation and the growth of microbes. Aim to keep your storage area cool, ideally between 60°F and 70°F. Also, protect your buds from direct sunlight. UV rays break down THC and other cannabinoids, weakening potency while increasing brittleness. Storing cannabis in opaque containers or dark spaces helps block light exposure, preserving both cannabinoid and terpene profiles.

Avoid cross-contamination by storing different strains and harvests separately. Mixing buds in one container might sound convenient, but it can introduce moisture and microbes from other batches. It can also muddle the unique flavors and aromas that make each strain special. Label your storage containers clearly and keep them separated. This practice not only maintains quality but also helps you track potency and cure progress more effectively.

When preparing cannabis for storage, ensure it has been properly dried and cured. Improperly dried buds retain excess moisture, creating an inviting environment for mold and bacteria. If you notice any soft, wet, or musty-smelling buds, avoid storing them immediately. Instead, allow them to dry further or cure properly before sealing them away. Remember, patience during drying and curing pays off in the long run with a safer, more potent product.

Storage containers should never be reused without proper cleaning. Even seemingly empty jars can harbor residual oils, contaminants, or spores from previous content. It's good practice to wash containers in warm, soapy water, rinse thoroughly, and dry completely before each use. For an added level of sterilization, rinsing with isopropyl alcohol and allowing the container to fully air dry can eliminate lingering microorganisms.

For growers storing cannabis over extended periods, routine inspections are necessary. Even with the best practices, sometimes conditions in storage can shift—for example, a container might develop slight moisture buildup due to fluctuating temperatures. Open your containers every week or so to check for signs of mold, mildew, or unusual odors. If you detect any contamination early, you can isolate affected buds and prevent it from spreading to the rest of your stash.

In addition to mold and bacteria, pests can also contaminate stored cannabis, though they're less common in sealed environments. Always ensure your grow and curing spaces remain pest-free to avoid hitchhikers making their way into your storage. Regularly clean the area around your storage containers and keep them elevated or sealed in pest-proof boxes if needed. Prevention at the source is key here. Once pests have infiltrated dried cannabis, elimination becomes difficult without degrading the product quality.

Many beginner growers underestimate the importance of airflow in preventing contamination during storage. While airtight containers are necessary, some level of controlled airflow is beneficial, especially during the curing phase which precedes final storage. If buds are placed into an airtight environment too early, residual moisture has nowhere to escape, leading to spoilage. During long-term storage, however, minimal airflow is better. Using containers with controlled resealing abilities, combined with humidity packs, strikes the right balance between preserving freshness and avoiding contamination.

Some growers also turn to vacuum sealing for cannabis storage, which removes air and reduces oxidation risk. While this can extend shelf life, vacuum sealing without proper humidity control can crush the buds or lock in moisture if they aren't perfectly dry. This causes mold risk to increase rather than decrease. It's vital to dry and cure thoroughly before vacuum sealing, and to combine this method with humidity control packets. Otherwise, vacuum sealing is best reserved for short-term transport or immediate use.

Avoid using storage containers or materials that emit chemicals or strong odors. Plastics that aren't food-grade can leach harmful substances into your cannabis over time. Likewise, wooden boxes or containers may contain resins or treatments that degrade the product or transfer tastes. Glass, ceramic, and high-quality metal containers generally present the safest options for cannabis storage.

Finally, it's critical to consider storage location in broader terms. Don't store cannabis near cleaning products, chemicals, or strong-smelling foods. Cannabis readily absorbs odors, compromising its natural aroma and flavor profiles. Storing cannabis in a dedicated, neutral-smelling area helps keep its true essence intact and prevents contamination by foreign smells or residues.

In summary, avoiding contamination in stored cannabis hinges on meticulous attention to cleanliness, environment, and handling. Use clean, airtight glass containers, maintain stable temperature and humidity, and handle buds with clean hands or gloves. Keep storage areas pest- and odor-free, maintain proper drying and curing before storage, and inspect your stash regularly. By weaving these precautions into your storage routine, you safeguard the hard work you put into cultivating quality cannabis, ensuring each bud stays fresh, flavorful, and safe for consumption.

CHAPTER 10
COMMON GROW PROBLEMS AND SOLUTIONS

Every grower, whether new or seasoned, runs into issues that can stall or ruin a cannabis crop if they're not spotted and handled quickly. Common problems include yellowing leaves, nutrient burn, pests, mold, and bud rot—all of which can stress your plants and reduce yield or potency. Understanding the signs early on sets you up for success: a few discolored leaves might mean a nutrient imbalance, while powdery spots could be mildew creeping in. Acting fast with the right adjustments—like tweaking feeding schedules, improving airflow, or using organic pest controls—can prevent small problems from turning into costly disasters. Staying attentive and learning to diagnose these challenges makes all the difference in growing healthy, vibrant plants that thrive through every stage.

Identifying Yellow Leaves, Bud Rot, and Nutrient Burn

As you progress in your cannabis cultivation journey, it's crucial to recognize common issues early on to prevent major setbacks. Among the most frequent problems growers face are yellow leaves, bud rot, and nutrient burn. These symptoms can look similar on the surface, but they stem from very different causes and require tailored solutions. Recognizing the subtle differences is the key to keeping your plants healthy and maximizing your harvest quality.

Let's start with yellow leaves, which is one of the most common visual cues that something's off with your plants. Yellowing, also known as chlorosis, often indicates an underlying nutritional or environmental problem. This symptom can appear as an overall yellow tint or as isolated yellow patches on the leaves. A telltale sign to watch for is whether the yellowing begins on the lower leaves and works its way up, or if it's concentrated punctually on newer growth. The progression can help you zero in on the root cause.

Yellow leaves could mean your cannabis is lacking essential nutrients, with nitrogen deficiency often being the first suspect. When nitrogen is in short supply, the plant cannibalizes it from older leaves to support new growth, causing those lower leaves to yellow and eventually die. However, yellowing doesn't always mean you need to add more nutrients. Sometimes it's about nutrient lockout, where the pH is off, preventing your plant from absorbing the nutrients already in the soil or growing medium. Properly checking and balancing pH can resolve this without throwing more fertilizer at the problem.

Environmental stressors play a big role too. Overwatering or underwatering can cause leaves to yellow and wilt, confusing many growers. Overwatering saturates the roots, cutting off oxygen and causing root rot, which leads to yellowing and drooping leaves. Conversely, underwatering dehydrates the plant, leading to yellow and dry foliage. Temperature extremes—whether too hot or cold—can also trigger leaf discoloration. Regular observation and maintaining a stable environment are vital to preventing these issues from snowballing.

Transitioning to bud rot, this is a nightmare scenario for flowering plants. Bud rot, or *Botrytis cinerea*, is a fungal pathogen that targets the dense flower buds where the moisture can get trapped. Early signs are subtle—a small brown or gray spot in the core of the bud that quickly spreads and causes the whole cluster to turn mushy and foul-smelling. Since bud rot loves humid conditions and poor airflow, it often surfaces in outdoor grows plagued with rain or in poorly ventilated indoor spaces.

Once bud rot takes hold, it spreads fast, especially during the late flowering stage when buds are heavy and densely packed. It's critical to inspect plants daily at this stage, breaking apart thick colas to check for hidden rot before it ruins your entire crop. Removing affected buds immediately and improving airflow can prevent the fungus from gaining ground. In serious cases, you might need to sacrifice some plants to save the rest.

Prevention is your best defense against bud rot. That means monitoring humidity levels, ideally keeping relative humidity between 40-50% during flowering. Using oscillating fans to circulate air and carefully pruning dense growth can open up the canopy and reduce moisture buildup. If you're growing outdoors, positioning plants to optimize sunlight and air circulation is essential.

Now, nutrient burn might seem like the opposite problem of deficiency, but it's just as common and equally damaging if ignored. Nutrient burn occurs when your plants receive too many nutrients, especially nitrogen, causing the leaf tips and edges to turn crisp and brown. It often looks like the tips are "burned" or burnt, and this condition can start in just a few days if you're feeding your plants aggressively.

One of the frustrating things about nutrient burn is how quickly it can develop and spread. If you don't catch it early, the damage pulls energy away from growth and bud development. Overfed plants can also become more vulnerable to pests and diseases because their stressed state weakens natural defenses. The best response is to flush your growing medium with clean, pH-balanced water to wash out excess fertilizers, then dial back your feeding schedule.

Recognizing nutrient burn isn't always straightforward, especially when compared to other nutrient issues. The crispy, darkened leaf tips are a hallmark, but you'll usually see this alongside an overall "frying" of leaf edges and sometimes twisting or curling leaves. The key difference between burn and deficiency is that with burn, yellowing and browning tend to start at the tips and edges, whereas deficiencies often begin in the leaf interior or on old vs. new growth depending on the nutrient.

It's also worth noting that a balanced feeding regime, tailored to your plant's life stage, is the best way to avoid both nutrient burn and deficiencies. Seedlings and young plants have different nutrient needs compared to mature flowering plants. Overestimating the power of nutrients or ignoring the specific requirements of your strain can easily lead to burn.

Summing up, learning to identify yellow leaves, bud rot, and nutrient burn boils down to careful observation and understanding the subtle signs unique to each condition. Each has distinct causes—nutrient shortage, fungal infection, and nutrient overdose respectively—and demands a different corrective approach. Armed with this knowledge, you'll be better prepared to respond quickly, protecting your plants and ensuring a successful harvest.

Next time you inspect your grow, take a close look at the leaf coloration, bud condition, and overall plant vigor. Question what could be causing any discoloration or rot and compare it against these common issues. Early detection is the difference between a minor fix and losing your crop to preventable problems. Taking proactive stepsâ from maintaining proper pH to managing humidity and feeding carefullyâ will reward you with healthier plants that thrive throughout their life cycle.

Recognizing and Managing Pests, Mold, and Mildew

One of the most frustrating challenges in cannabis cultivation is dealing with pests, mold, and mildew. These issues can sneak up on you quickly and, if left unchecked, can ruin your entire crop. Recognizing the warning signs early and knowing how to handle them effectively is critical to keeping your plants healthy and thriving. Every grower, whether new or seasoned, needs a solid grasp on identifying common invaders and diseases that threaten cannabis plants.

Pests like spider mites, aphids, thrips, and fungus gnats are frequent offenders in the grow room or garden. These tiny creatures feed on your plants, potentially spreading viruses or triggering stress responses that stunt growth. Spider mites, for instance, leave tiny yellow or white spots on leaves and spin webs that can coat entire sections of your plant. Aphids often cluster on the undersides of leaves, sucking sap and secreting sticky honeydew that attracts mold. Muskier insects like thrips can cause silvery streaks or speckling, while fungus gnats mostly become a problem in overly moist soil, where larvae feast on roots.

It's essential to inspect your plants regularly, paying special attention to the leaves—both tops and bottoms—as well as the stems and soil surface. A magnifying glass or a jeweler's loupe can help you get a better look at tiny invaders. Catching pests early is your best bet for limiting damage. Left to multiply, they can quickly overwhelm your crop. Aside from visible damage, signs like yellowing leaves, curled or distorted growth, and weakened plants can all hint that pests are undermining your efforts.

On the fungal side, mold and mildew are equally notorious for wreaking havoc. Powdery mildew forms a white, dusty coating on leaves and buds and thrives in environments with poor airflow and high humidity. Botrytis, often called bud rot, is a devastating mold that can destroy flowers from the inside out, turning them into soft, gray mush. These fungi are opportunistic and love taking advantage of humid, crowded conditions and plants with dense buds where air movement is limited.

Preventing mold and mildew starts with managing your grow environment. Good airflow, consistent temperature control, and keeping humidity levels in check during flowering are foundational steps. Use fans and ventilation to keep the air moving and avoid overcrowding your plants, which creates pockets of stagnant, moist air. Monitoring humidity closely—aiming for 40-50% during flowering—can drastically reduce your risk.

Managing pests and pathogens often requires an integrated approach. Relying on a single solution rarely brings lasting results. Start by maintaining cleanliness in your grow space. Regularly sanitize your tools, pots, and work surfaces. Avoid bringing in outside contaminants on your clothing, tools, or new plants. Quarantining any new additions for a week or two before introducing them to your main crop can prevent pest hitchhikers.

When it comes to direct treatment, organic and biological control methods provide effective, safe options that keep your cannabis healthy without harmful chemicals. Beneficial insects such as ladybugs, predatory mites, and nematodes can be excellent allies. Ladybugs consume aphids and small pests, while predatory mites target spider mites and thrips. Nematodes, microscopic roundworms, can help control fungus gnat larvae in the soil.

In cases where pest infestations grow beyond manageable levels, neem oil sprays or insecticidal soaps are practical tools. Neem oil works well against many pests and also has antifungal properties, making it a versatile option. However, it's vital to apply such treatments carefully, ideally during vegetation stages or early flowering, and always follow product guidelines.

Avoid spraying oils directly onto buds late in flowering to preserve quality and avoid residue.

Mold and mildew often require a more aggressive response, especially if detected during flowering. Removing and discarding infected buds immediately helps to slow or stop the spread. For powdery mildew, several fungicides are available, but growers often prefer sulfur or potassium bicarbonate treatments because they're less harsh and safer for cannabis. Maintaining strict environmental control remains the most effective ongoing solution against these fungal threats.

Sometimes, despite best efforts, pests or mold outbreaks will happen. When that occurs, don't get discouraged. Treat the problem quickly, adjust your environmental controls, and monitor plants intensively in the days following treatment. Remember, prevention is easier and less costly than eradication. Establishing solid routines for inspection, sanitation, and environmental management will reduce your risk and help you catch trouble before it spreads.

Keeping a detailed grow journal proves invaluable when managing these issues. Recording observations about pest presence, humidity levels, plant health, and any treatments applied helps track effectiveness and identify recurring weak points in your system. Over time, this data lets you fine-tune your approach and avoid repeating the same mistakes. Whether growing indoors or outdoors, consistency and vigilance are your best friends.

Additionally, understanding that some pest presence is normal helps maintain realistic expectations. Complete eradication isn't always possible or necessary—aim instead for control and balance. Healthy plants can often outgrow minor pest damage, especially if their environment supports robust growth and immunity. Keeping plants well-nourished and stress-free strengthens their natural defenses against both pests and disease.

In outdoor grows, pest and mold pressures can be more unpredictable. You need to adjust strategies based on season, climate, and local insect populations. Natural predators tend to be more abundant outdoors, which can help, but weather changes may also spur sudden fungal growth or insect hatches. Scout plants frequently and prepare to intervene sooner if you see signs of trouble. Row spacings that allow sunlight and airflow to penetrate the canopy reduce many hazards common to outdoor cultivation.

Ultimately, recognizing and managing pests, mold, and mildew is about being proactive, hands-on, and observant. No matter your experience level, regular plant inspections combined with environmental controls and non-toxic treatments create a strong defense. Addressing problems early not only protects your crop but also keeps your growing process more enjoyable and rewarding.

Healthy plants are happy plants—and happy plants produce the best buds.

How to Diagnose Problems and Respond Quickly

Every grower, no matter how experienced, eventually encounters issues with their cannabis plants. The key to maintaining healthy crops and achieving great yields lies in the ability to spot problems early and respond swiftly before minor issues turn into major setbacks. Diagnosing problems effectively starts with vigilance—regularly inspecting your plants, your environment, and your equipment to catch any signs that something is out of balance.

One of the most important habits you can develop as a grower is daily observation. Inconsistencies often appear slowly and subtly at first: a tiny yellow spot on a leaf, a slight curling at the edges, or a change in stem color. These small clues are your plants' way of communicating stress, deficiency, or disease. By training yourself to recognize these early warning signs, you give yourself a crucial advantage in maintaining a healthy grow.

When you notice something unusual, don't panic. Instead, take a systematic and calm approach to diagnose the issue. Start by gathering as much information as possible. Consider your plant's recent care routine—have you changed the nutrient schedule or watering frequency? Is there been a fluctuation in temperature or humidity in your grow space? Any alterations in environmental factors often trigger problems, so reviewing recent changes is an excellent first step.

Next, examine different parts of the plant closely. Look at the leaves, stems, and buds for discoloration, spots, or deformation. Check the soil or growing medium as well—dryness, waterlogging, or unusual smells can also hint at underlying issues. Pest presence should not be overlooked either: inspect the undersides of leaves and the growing medium for insects, eggs, or webs. These pests not only drain plant vigor but can spread diseases rapidly if left unchecked.

Once you've identified the symptoms, try to narrow down the potential causes. Many cannabis problems share overlapping signs, making diagnosis tricky without context. For example, yellowing leaves might signal nutrient deficiencies, overwatering, root-bound conditions, or pest damage, depending on the bigger picture. That's why cross-referencing symptoms with your environmental conditions and treatment history is vital.

There are a few key categories of cannabis problems to keep in mind: nutrient imbalances, water-related stress, pest infestations, and environmental factors like temperature or humidity extremes. It's helpful to remember that these categories often interplay. Overwatering can lead to root rot, humidity spikes can invite mold, and deficiencies can weaken plants, leaving them open to pest attacks.

Rapid response is essential once you've confirmed the problem. Waiting too long only allows issues to escalate, making recovery more difficult and sometimes impossible. For example, if you detect early signs of nutrient burn, flushing the grow medium with clean, pH-balanced water can prevent damage from worsening. If pests are spotted, introducing biological controls or safe insecticides immediately limits population growth. In every case, speed combined with targeted action increases your chances of saving affected plants.

Logging all your observations and treatments is a practical approach that pays off in the long run. By keeping a detailed grow journal, you'll begin to notice patterns and improve your diagnosis accuracy over time. Note everything from watering schedules to lighting changes, temperatures, humidity levels, and any issues that arise alongside your corrective measures. This record becomes an invaluable reference for troubleshooting future problems and fine-tuning your grow process.

Sometimes, problems won't be straightforward, and you might encounter symptoms that don't fit common scenarios. In those moments, it's useful to tap into the wider cannabis growing community. Forums, grower groups, and trusted online resources can offer guidance, fresh perspectives, or even identify rare problems based on your descriptions and photos. Don't hesitate to seek advice; collaboration is one of the fastest routes to resolution.

One big challenge in diagnosing cannabis problems is staying objective and avoiding assumptions. It's tempting to jump to conclusions—like blaming pests for every leaf discoloration—but a disconnected approach rarely fixes the real issue. Systematic testing and ruling out causes one step at a time will get you to the root problem quicker. Using control tests, like adjusting one variable per cycle, helps minimize guesswork and clarify cause-effect relationships.

Visual aids such as charts, leaf guides, or mobile apps designed to identify nutrient deficiencies or pest damage can be handy tools to enhance your diagnosis process. While these tools shouldn't replace hands-on observation, they provide helpful starting points—especially for beginners still learning the plant's language.

Speed does not mean rushing carelessly, though. Quick responses should always be well-informed. Wild adjustments—like doubling nutrients or using harsh chemicals without proper identification—might cause more harm than good. Instead, prioritize gradual corrections and monitor closely to see how your plants respond. If uncertain, err on the side of caution and focus on optimizing basic environmental factors like lighting, airflow, and watering, which play a foundational role in health.

In summary, effective diagnosis and quick reaction demand a combination of regular observation, methodical evaluation, clear record-keeping, and thoughtful intervention. This cycle—spotting the issue, analyzing symptoms, pinpointing causes, then acting promptly—is the backbone of successful cannabis cultivation. With practice, you'll get faster, more accurate with diagnosis, and your plants will thrive better despite the inevitable growing challenges along the way.

Remember, problems don't have to be setbacks; they're learning opportunities. Each time you diagnose and solve an issue, you build knowledge and confidence. That resilience is what transforms good growers into great cultivators capable of producing high-quality cannabis consistently, no matter what arises in the grow room.

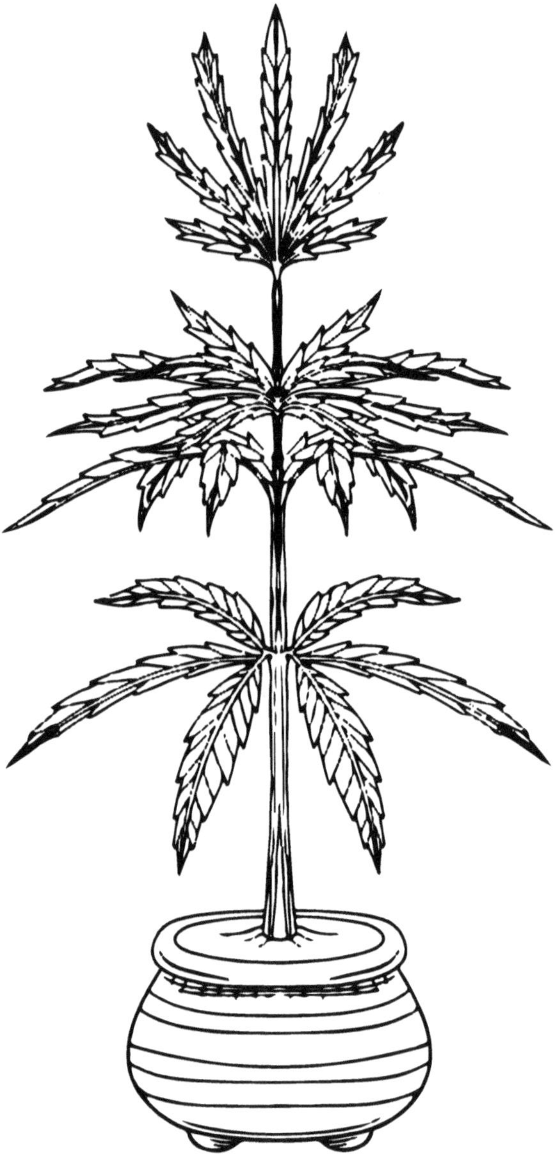

CHAPTER 11
BOOSTING YIELDS AND POTENCY

Unlocking the full potential of your cannabis plants involves a blend of smart techniques and consistent care, aimed at both quantity and quality. Enhancing yields isn't just about pushing your plants harder, but about understanding their needs and responding with precision—whether that means optimizing light intensity, introducing controlled pruning to encourage growth, or adjusting environmental factors like CO_2 levels to accelerate photosynthesis. Potency improves when plants are less stressed and grown in nutrient-rich, organic soils that help lock in flavors and cannabinoids naturally. Many experienced growers swear by combining these elements thoughtfully, creating an environment where plants can thrive and truly express their genetic potential, ultimately rewarding your efforts with bigger, more potent buds that stand out in any grow operation.

Using CO2, Pruning, and Advanced Lighting Techniques

When it comes to boosting your cannabis yields and potency, three powerful tools stand out: enriching your grow space with CO2, implementing strategic pruning methods, and utilizing advanced lighting technology. Each of these elements plays a critical role in enhancing plant growth and resin production, and when combined thoughtfully, they can transform an average harvest into an exceptional one. This section will walk you through how these factors interact and how to effectively integrate them into your cultivation routine.

Let's start with carbon dioxide, or CO2. While we naturally think of air as the perfect environment for plants, they actually thrive when CO2 levels are elevated beyond what's typically found outdoors. Standard atmospheric CO2 hovers around 400 parts per million (ppm), but cannabis plants can use carbon dioxide efficiently up to about 1,200 to 1,500 ppm in controlled environments. Adding CO2 to your grow space accelerates photosynthesis, allowing the plants to produce more sugars and energy to fuel robust growth and bigger buds.

Using supplemental CO2 is most effective when combined with optimal light intensity. Plants can only make use of extra CO2 if their lighting supports an increased rate of photosynthesis. Typically, this means employing high-quality HID lights like High-Pressure Sodium (HPS) or Metal Halide, or full-spectrum LED systems that deliver intense, targeted light across the spectrum cannabis plants need. Without adequate light, raising CO2 won't provide noticeable benefits and can even waste resources. So before investing in CO2, make sure your lighting setup is rock solid.

One of the biggest reasons growers hesitate with CO2 is the complexity involved. You'll need a system to monitor and control CO2 levels accurately—too much can be harmful, too little won't make a difference. Beginners might consider simple CO2 bags or passive generators initially, which release CO2 gradually without electronic controllers. More advanced cultivators can step up to pressurized CO2 tanks paired with regulators and digital controllers that keep concentrations steady. Whichever approach you choose, timing matters. Enriching CO2 during the daytime when lights are on is crucial since plants only photosynthesize in the light. Shutting off supplemental CO2 at night saves resources and maintains a natural environment for your plants.

Now, moving on to pruning—it's a practice experienced growers swear by for increasing both yield and potency. Effective pruning doesn't just clear out unwanted growth; it's about sculpting your plants for maximum light penetration and airflow. This encourages your cannabis to develop more flowering sites and reduces issues with mold or pests by keeping buds dry and healthy.

One popular pruning technique is removing lower branches and small growth that won't get enough light to mature properly. These "sucker" branches consume energy but rarely produce quality buds. Taking them off early in the flowering phase redirects the plant's energy to the bigger colas receiving prime light. Another crucial aspect is "defoliation," carefully trimming excess leaves blocking light from reaching bud sites underneath the canopy. While it might seem like you're sacrificing growth, you're actually improving overall efficiency and bud development.

Pruning also works hand-in-hand with training methods like topping or low-stress training, but it's important to prune thoughtfully. Over-pruning can stress your plants and stunt growth; timing is everything. The best time to prune is usually during the late vegetative phase or early flowering when removing certain leaves and branches won't negatively impact flowering or yield. Watch your plants closely and only prune what's necessary to optimize airflow and light distribution.

In addition to CO2 and pruning, lighting techniques have come a long way and can drastically influence your final harvest. Gone are the days when a simple light bulb sufficed. Growers now have access to an array of lighting styles designed to meet specific cannabis growth needs while reducing energy consumption and heat output.

LED technology, for example, has revolutionized how many home growers approach lighting. Full-spectrum LED grow lights provide a mix of red, blue, and sometimes ultraviolet light tailored precisely to cannabis plants' photosynthetic requirements. They produce less heat compared to traditional HPS lamps, allowing your grow environment to stay cooler and reducing the risk of heat stress. LEDs also let you position lights closer to your canopy without burning your plants, which enhances light intensity and penetration.

However, High-Pressure Sodium (HPS) lights still hold a respected place in flowering stages. Their strong red and orange light spectrum encourages dense bud formation, often producing bigger yields. Some growers even combine HPS with Metal Halide (MH) lights or switch between these to mimic natural seasonal light changes. Another exciting option is Ceramic Metal Halide (CMH) lighting, which offers a fuller spectrum and longer bulb life compared to traditional HPS or MH lights.

Beyond the type of light, the way you deliver and manage that light during your cannabis cycle is equally important. Adjusting light height and intensity ensures even canopy coverage, preventing some buds from becoming underdeveloped "shade" zones. As your plants grow taller, it's crucial to raise lights systematically to maintain the optimal distance—usually between 12 to 24 inches depending on the light's wattage and type—and prevent heat damage or light burn.

Using reflective materials in your grow room or tent can also improve lighting efficiency dramatically.

Reflective walls bounce stray light back onto your plants, meaning fewer watts are wasted. Reflective mylar or white walls are popular for their high reflectance and durability. Maximizing your light's output this way can increase photosynthesis and bud growth without additional electricity costs.

Implementing advanced lighting schedules also helps improve potency and yields. While the foundational schedule of 18 hours light/6 hours dark in vegetative growth and 12/12 in flowering remain standard, some growers experiment with light interruptions or gradual adjustments to smooth the transition into flowering. These subtle tweaks can sometimes reduce plant stress and increase cannabinoid production, though results may vary based on strain and environment.

Integrating CO2, pruning, and advanced lighting might sound a bit intimidating at first, but when done with patience and observation, the rewards are substantial. Plants respond visibly to better air quality, improved light, and thoughtful canopy management. You'll notice stronger branches, more abundant and evenly developed buds, and richer resin production that directly correlates with potency. Keep in mind, balance is key—each aspect complements the others, but none functions effectively in isolation.

If you're just getting started, consider introducing each element one at a time. Begin by upgrading your lighting to a full-spectrum LED or enhancing your existing setup's efficiency with reflectors. Once your lighting is dialed in, experiment with pruning practices tailored to your strain's growth habits. Finally, introduce CO2 enrichment as a final step in your optimization process to give plants that extra push during peak growth.

Growing cannabis isn't just about following a recipe; it's about learning how each environmental factor shapes your plants. Using supplemental CO2 promotes photosynthesis and energy production, pruning shapes your plants for airflow and light access, and advanced lighting techniques provide the precise power cannabis needs to thrive. When you add these together, you're laying the foundation for significantly bigger and more potent buds.

The journey to a successful and bountiful grow requires attention, adjustment, and sometimes a little experimentation. Keep logs of your setups and results, so you can refine your approach each time. Over multiple cycles, these enhancements will become second nature, and the quality of your cannabis will reflect your dedication. Elevated CO2 levels, intelligent pruning, and cutting-edge lighting—master these well, and your harvests will thank you handsomely.

Organic Growing Techniques and Super Soils Explained

When aiming to boost both yield and potency, one of the most rewarding approaches is embracing organic growing techniques combined with super soils. These methods not only promote healthier plants but also naturally enhance flavor, aroma, and cannabinoid profiles without relying heavily on synthetic inputs. For anyone looking to achieve exceptional results while keeping their grow environmentally friendly, understanding organic cultivation and the magic behind super soils is a crucial step.

Organic growing starts with the soil—it really is the foundation of plant health. Unlike conventional methods that use chemical nutrients, organic growing encourages a thriving ecosystem within the soil, full of beneficial microbes, fungi, and earthworms. These living organisms break down organic matter into nutrients plants can absorb easily. This natural nutrient cycling not only sustains the cannabis plant but also produces robust root systems and vigorous vegetative growth. When plants build a strong root network, they naturally produce more resins and terpenes, resulting in higher potency.

What distinguishes organic growing is the focus on feeding the soil, rather than directly feeding the plant. Many growers find this approach develops healthier plants that can better resist pests and diseases, decreasing the need for harsh pesticides. Over time, organic soils improve in structure and fertility, meaning each successive grow benefits from richer, more life-filled earth. This evolution creates a self-sustaining environment that supports abundant, high-quality cannabis yields.

Super soils take organic growing one step further. They consist of carefully mixed ingredients, often a blend of composts, worm castings, bat guano, rock dust minerals, biochar, and various organic amendments. This mixture is designed to provide all essential nutrients throughout the plant's life cycle, eliminating—or significantly reducing—the need for additional feeding.

The beauty of super soil lies in its ability to release nutrients slowly and steadily. This slow-release nutrient profile mimics natural soil behavior found in wild ecosystems, where plants thrive on a continuous supply of nourishment made available by microbial activity. When growing cannabis in super soil, the roots can explore an inviting environment saturated with beneficial organisms and rich in diverse nutrition. This leads to slower, steadier growth and ultimately more resinous and flavorful buds.

One key to creating super soil is balancing the carbon-to-nitrogen (C:N) ratio. High-carbon materials such as peat moss, coconut coir, or composted wood chips provide energy sources for microbes, while nitrogen-rich amendments like alfalfa meal or blood meal offer essential nutrients for plant growth. Achieving the right ratio encourages microbial activity that converts organic compounds into plant-available forms. A well-balanced super soil typically includes mineral amendments, such as dolomite lime to adjust pH and basalt rock dust for trace minerals. These minerals are often overlooked but play a vital role in supporting enzyme functions and overall plant metabolism.

After mixing, the soil is typically "cooked" or aged for a few weeks. This process allows microbes to break down the organic matter fully, stabilizes nutrient availability, and prevents burning sensitive plants with excess ammonia or nitrogen spikes. During this time, temperature and moisture levels should be monitored carefully to support balanced microbial activity. Once mature, this super soil becomes a living, breathing medium ready to deliver nutrients organically and efficiently.

Besides nutrient delivery, organic and super soils foster a unique synergy in the root zone. Beneficial bacteria and mycorrhizal fungi form symbiotic relationships with cannabis roots, expanding their reach and ability to absorb water and nutrients effectively. These relationships enhance plant stress tolerance, facilitating better recovery from environmental stressors such as temperature fluctuations or mild drought. For growers seeking to maximize their garden's natural resilience, nurturing these relationships through organic methods is invaluable.

Another notable advantage of organic growing is the improvement in flavor and aroma that many cultivators swear by. Synthetic fertilizers can sometimes produce fast growth but may leave the final product tasting harsher or less complex. On the other hand, nutrients delivered naturally within super soils tend to highlight a cannabis strain's full terpene profile. This complexity elevates the smoking or vaping experience, making the extra time and effort to prepare super soils worthwhile.

While creating and using super soils might seem daunting at first, the potential payoff is well worth the effort. The process also aligns closely with sustainable and eco-conscious growing practices because it minimizes runoff and chemical use. For growers keen on reducing their environmental footprint, organic techniques represent an increasingly popular path. Plus, the knowledge that your cannabis is grown with natural methods can bring some added satisfaction alongside a superior final product.

It's worth noting that organic growing requires patience and observation. Plants may not explode in height as quickly as with synthetic feeds, but they tend to develop sturdier structures and resin glands packed deeper with cannabinoids. Many veteran growers report a lasting quality in their harvests that synthetic methods fail to replicate. That means organic isn't just about ideology—it's about recognizing what produces the best cannabis in both potency and experience.

One common challenge is maintaining the right environment for microbial life. Soil temperature, moisture, and pH all need to be between specific ranges to encourage beneficial organisms to thrive. For example, soils kept too wet can become anaerobic, starving useful microbes of oxygen. Growers must strike a balance with watering practices here—neither too dry nor too saturated. Adding mulch or organic ground cover can help regulate moisture and temperature, supporting the soil biome throughout the growing season.

In addition, organic growers often incorporate compost teas or microbial inoculants as supplements to boost the life in their super soils. These teas introduce beneficial bacteria and fungi actively into the root zone, especially during critical growth stages. They can improve nutrient uptake, reduce disease prevalence, and increase root mass, all contributing to thicker, more potent buds. While not strictly necessary if your super soil is well-made, these additions can accelerate or reinforce the natural processes already at work.

Understanding that organic grows are inherently slower and more deliberate can be a mindset shift but one that is rewarding. This style of cultivation emphasizes respect for natural rhythms rather than pushing plants aggressively with chemical fertilizers and additives. It's a holistic art as much as a science, combining soil biology with attentive plant care to coax the best from your crop.

To summarize, organic growing techniques and super soils form a powerful foundation for anyone interested in boosting yields and potency naturally. By fostering a living soil ecosystem brimming with nutrients and beneficial organisms, growers can produce cannabis that's not only bountiful but also rich in terpene and cannabinoid complexity. The process requires planning and patience but repays with superior quality, healthier plants, and a more sustainable way to cultivate cannabis at home. Whether you're a beginner eager to grow your first batch or an experienced cultivator aiming to elevate your garden, diving into organic methods and super soils offers a pathway to truly exceptional results.

Tips and Tricks from Experienced Commercial Growers

When it comes to boosting your cannabis yields and potency, tapping into the wealth of knowledge from commercial growers can make a world of difference. These seasoned cultivators have spent years honing their craft and optimizing every aspect of the grow cycle. While home growers might not have the exact scale or budget of a commercial grow operation, many techniques and mindsets they follow translate well to smaller setups. Understanding these tips often means thinking beyond the basics and embracing a more meticulous, detail-oriented approach.

One of the biggest lessons commercial growers emphasize is the importance of consistency. They know that cannabis plants thrive best when their environment is stable and predictable. Instead of overreacting to every minor change or challenge, they focus on controlling key variables like temperature, humidity, and nutrient delivery with as much precision as possible. That mindset prevents stress on the plants, which can negatively affect both yield and cannabinoid production. It's worth noting that this doesn't mean obsessiveness; rather, it's about building a routine and sticking to it, making adjustments only when there is clear evidence something is off.

Another critical piece of wisdom from experienced growers is the way they view pruning and training. While younger growers might shy away from topping or super cropping due to fear of damaging the plant, commercial cultivators understand that strategic stress can lead to more vigorous growth and bigger buds. They carefully prune lower branches and less productive growth to redirect the plant's energy into its top colas. The result is not just higher yield but often better-quality buds packed with trichomes. Learning to read your plants' responses and timing these techniques just right is something that comes with experience, but once mastered, it becomes a powerful tool in your arsenal.

Lighting is another area where commercial expertise shines through. These growers don't just rely on turning lights on and off; they invest time into understanding the precise spectrum and intensity that works best for different growth stages. For example, they adjust light spectrums to favor blue wavelengths during vegetative phases to encourage bushier growth, then switch to more red-dominant spectrums during flowering to boost bud development. Modulating light intensity to match the plants' maturation also prevents light burn and optimizes photosynthesis. While this may sound complex, even small adjustments—like raising or lowering your lights depending on plant response—can have big benefits.

One overlooked trick from commercial operations involves air circulation and CO2 enrichment. These growers know that stale air can lead to lower yields and weaker potency because it inhibits the plants' ability to photosynthesize efficiently. Even if you can't afford a CO2 generator, ensuring proper air exchange and ventilation goes a long way. Fans placed strategically help simulate natural wind, strengthening stems and reducing the risk of mold. For those who are ready to take it a step further, supplemental CO2 during peak light hours can increase growth rates and final bud density, but only if other factors like light and nutrients are dialed in properly.

Soil and nutrients also get a premium in commercial setups. Experienced growers often prefer organic or super soil blends that support a rich microbiome, which helps plants access nutrients more effectively and organically fend off pests and diseases. They're careful not to overfeed at any stage; instead, they watch how their plants react and adjust inputs as needed. Overfeeding is one of the top mistakes that can compromise not only yield but the flavor and potency of the final product. Patience and observation become crucial here—good growers learn to "feed the soil, not just the plant."

Watering techniques deserve a nod as well. Many commercial growers swear by a strict watering schedule paired with frequent checks of soil moisture levels. They avoid the temptation to water on a set timetable regardless of plant needs and instead learn to recognize the signals—drooping leaves, dryness or excessive wetness in the medium. Proper watering encourages deep root growth, which underpins healthy, resilient plants that ultimately produce more potent flowers. Runoff testing is another habit they adopt to catch nutrient imbalances early, something home growers can implement with little cost.

Environmental monitoring is an area where experienced growers pull ahead by leveraging technology. Most commercial facilities use digital sensors to continuously track temperature, humidity, CO2 levels, and light cycles. This data-driven approach means issues get caught quickly and conditions remain ideal. While full automation may be beyond many home growers, using affordable hygrometers and thermometers to get detailed feedback is an easy step. Keeping a grow journal or digital log to record changes, observations, and results can also mimic the professional approach and help refine your methods over time.

One subtle but important trick is managing plant density and spacing. Experienced commercial cultivators avoid overcrowding, which can suffocate lower branches and create microclimates ripe for mold and pests. They train their plants apart enough to allow for good airflow and light penetration. Thinning out weaker plants or cutting back excessive fan leaves ensures energy goes toward the biggest tops and helps produce denser buds with better cannabinoid content. This isn't about sacrificing quantity, but about quality control through intelligent cultivation strategies.

Experienced growers keep a long-term perspective, focusing on soil health and sustainability to maintain productivity year after year. They avoid quick fixes, instead building their grow medium and environment to support each cannabis cycle holistically—from seedling to harvest and beyond. Understanding that cannabis is a living organism that interacts with its environment encourages growers to nurture their plants carefully instead of rushing every step. This approach may seem slower upfront, but it pays off in more potent, flavorful, and higher-yielding harvests.

Picking the right strain and matching it with your grow environment is something commercial growers have down to a science. While it's easy to get distracted by flashy genetics, smart cultivators choose varieties known for stability and vigor under their specific conditions. This ensures predictable results and less frustration. Over time, they map which strains respond best to certain nutrients, lighting, or training methods and build around those proven winners. Home growers might find experimenting with a couple of stable strains before trying rarer genetics can optimize their success.

Finally, experienced commercial growers emphasize ongoing education and community. They know that trends and techniques evolve, and staying connected to forums, workshops, or local grower groups provides fresh insights. Sharing successes and failures helps everyone improve. Approaching your grow with curiosity and a willingness to adjust your methods based on new information keeps you growing alongside your plants. Success in cannabis cultivation is rarely about one giant breakthrough—it's about small improvements and keen attention paid consistently over time.

Bringing these tips into your own grow, no matter the size or budget, means adopting a mindset of care, precision, and observation. Commercial growers focus on enhancing every detail, from air circulation to nutrient balance to training techniques, all to unlock their plants' fullest potential. By applying these strategies with the right amount of patience and experimentation, you'll find that boosting yields and potency isn't just a commercial secret—it can be your home-grown reality.

Chapter 12
Growing Sustainably and Legally

As you expand your cannabis cultivation journey, focusing on sustainable and legal practices isn't just smart—it ensures your grows thrive without causing harm to the environment or putting you at risk legally. Embracing eco-friendly methods, like conserving water and choosing organic inputs, helps maintain a healthy balance between your garden and the planet. Equally important is staying informed about the local and state laws that govern cannabis growing, since compliance not only protects you from penalties but also supports the broader acceptance of home cultivation. Growing responsibly means respecting community guidelines while implementing ethical approaches that set a positive example for other cultivators, ultimately creating a future where high-quality cannabis is grown with care and respect for both nature and the law.

Eco-Friendly Cannabis Cultivation Practices

Growing cannabis responsibly means more than just following legal guidelines—it also means caring for the environment and minimizing your ecological footprint. In recent years, the cannabis industry has grown rapidly, often consuming large amounts of water, electricity, and other resources. As a home cultivator aiming to elevate your grow, adopting eco-friendly practices isn't just good for the planet—it actually helps improve the health and quality of your plants, too. By integrating sustainability into your routine, you not only protect the environment but also build a more resilient and cost-effective garden.

One of the foundations of eco-friendly cultivation is efficient resource use. Cannabis plants can be thirsty, but that doesn't mean you have to waste water. Collecting rainwater or harvesting greywater (water that's been lightly used around the house) can reduce the need for fresh water. Using drip irrigation systems or soaker hoses delivers water directly to the plant roots, significantly cutting down on run-off and evaporation. By watering only what's necessary and at the right times of day, you conserve vital water resources and keep your plants healthier, as overwatering can lead to root rot and other issues.

Energy consumption is another critical area. Indoor cultivation setups often rely on high-intensity lighting and ventilation systems, which can consume a lot of electricity. Switching to energy-efficient LED lights is one of the most effective ways to reduce power use. LEDs produce less heat compared to traditional HID lamps, meaning your grow room requires less cooling, which in turn means less energy spent running fans or air conditioners. Many modern LEDs are adjustable, letting you fine-tune the light spectrum for different growth stages, which can improve yields while saving power.

For outdoor growers, the key to sustainability lies in working with nature rather than against it. Choosing a site with good sunlight exposure and natural drainage reduces the need for artificial lighting or pumping water. Using organic mulch helps retain soil moisture and suppress weeds, which cuts down on watering and eliminates the need for chemical herbicides. Plus, mulch adds nutrients back into the soil as it breaks down, enhancing plant growth naturally. Strategically planting native companion plants can improve soil health, deter pests, and encourage beneficial insects, creating a balanced mini-ecosystem around your cannabis plants.

Speaking of soil, going organic is one of the most impactful changes a grower can make for sustainability. Synthetic fertilizers and pesticides might boost plant growth short-term, but they can harm beneficial soil microbes, contaminate water sources, and leave chemical residues. Organic soil amendments—such as compost, worm castings, bat guano, and mycorrhizal fungi—nurture the soil's microbial life, which helps plants absorb nutrients more efficiently and resist disease naturally.

Composting your plant waste and other biodegradable kitchen scraps turns what would be garbage into valuable soil feed, reducing landfill waste and fostering a circular system in your garden.

Another important consideration is pest management. Avoid using harsh chemical pesticides which can disrupt local wildlife and reduce beneficial insect populations. Instead, opt for integrated pest management (IPM) techniques—combining preventative measures, biological controls like ladybugs or predatory mites, and organic sprays only when absolutely necessary. Encouraging a healthy ecosystem around your grow space lets nature take care of many pest problems on its own. Regular scouting and early detection make it easier to control pests before they damage your crop or require drastic measures.

Waste reduction plays a vital role as well. Many growers overlook how much plastic, packaging, and non-biodegradable materials are used during cultivation. By choosing reusable pots, containers, and trays made from sustainable materials, you minimize single-use waste. Reusing or repurposing old equipment extends their life and keeps them out of the landfill. When possible, buy supplies in bulk to reduce packaging, and recycle plastics and paper responsibly. Even trimming scraps and damaged plant material can be composted instead of tossed.

Temperature and humidity control also affect your ecological footprint. Overcooling or overheating not only raises energy bills but stresses plants, potentially leading to lower yields. Investing in smart climate control tools and sensors allows you to maintain optimal conditions efficiently. Implementing shading techniques or ventilation improvements can lessen the need for electrical cooling. For outdoor growers, planning planting schedules around local climate cycles reduces the chances of extreme temperature stress, cutting down on water and energy inputs.

Another forward-thinking approach involves exploring renewable energy sources. Solar panels or small wind turbines can help offset electricity used in indoor grows, especially for dedicated enthusiasts who want to achieve a carbon-neutral operation. While the initial investment may seem steep, incentives and rebates in many regions make these systems more affordable than ever. Over time, green energy pays off by lowering power costs and reducing reliance on fossil fuels.

Finally, staying informed about sustainability trends and advances empowers you to continuously improve your grow. Regulations and technology in cannabis cultivation evolve quickly, opening doors to innovative eco-friendly products and practices. Networking with other responsible growers, attending workshops, and reading up-to-date resources keeps your knowledge fresh and your garden thriving without compromising the planet.

Making small, practical changes in your growing routine can create a substantial positive impact. Whether it's switching to drip irrigation, adopting organic nutrients, or upgrading lighting to LEDs, each step reduces your environmental footprint and supports healthier plants. Embracing eco-friendly cannabis cultivation is not just a trend—it's becoming a standard for growers who want to enjoy high-quality cannabis today while ensuring the earth stays vibrant for future harvests.

By nourishing the environment as you cultivate, you cultivate success on multiple levels. The healthier your soil, the better your plants will thrive; the smarter your water use, the stronger your crop; the more mindful your energy consumption, the more sustainable your grow becomes. This synergy between nature and nurture sets the stage for a rewarding cannabis growing experience that's good for you, your community, and the planet.

Navigating Local and State Cannabis Laws

When stepping into the world of home cannabis cultivation, understanding the maze of local and state laws isn't just a good idea—it's an absolute necessity. Laws around cannabis can differ wildly, not only from state to state but even between cities or counties within the same state. This patchwork of regulations affects how, when, and where you can legally grow cannabis, making it crucial to get up to speed before you plant your first seed. Ignoring legal guidelines can lead to serious consequences, from hefty fines to criminal charges. Staying informed and compliant is key to cultivating cannabis safely and sustainably.

One of the first things to keep in mind is that cannabis laws generally revolve around a few main points: how many plants you can grow, where you can grow them, and who is allowed to participate in cultivation. Most states that permit personal cultivation set a maximum number of plants per household or per adult. These limits can range significantly—from as few as two or four plants to a dozen or more. Some states distinguish between mature and immature plants as well, often allowing a larger number of seedlings or clones but restricting the count of flowering, mature plants. Exceeding these limits, even accidentally, can put a grower at risk of legal trouble.

Additionally, many laws place restrictions on the visibility and security of your grow operation. For instance, some states require cannabis plants to be out of public view, meaning you can't have a garden visible from the street or a neighbor's property. Others insist on secure enclosures to prevent unauthorized access, which is especially important if you live with children or in a shared housing environment. Knowing the specifics here helps protect your privacy and reduces the chances of complaints or investigations.

It also pays to be mindful of zoning rules and local ordinances. Even if state law permits growing cannabis, municipalities may impose their own restrictions that affect where you're allowed to grow. Some cities ban home cultivation entirely, while others regulate it heavily, including rules about odor control, lighting, or the use of pesticides and fertilizers. This means that what's legal in one part of a state might be illegal just a few miles away. Checking with local government websites, city ordinances, or local cannabis compliance offices can help untangle these nuances.

Another important angle lies in residency and age requirements. While most states require growers to be at least 21 years old, some have additional residency stipulations for cultivating cannabis at home. In some places, only state residents or those who have lived in the state for a certain period qualify to grow legally. Visitors or temporary residents might not have the same rights to cultivate, so this is vital for anyone who moves frequently or is considering growing while away from their permanent home.

Beyond individual cultivation, there are also distinctions between medical and recreational cannabis laws. If you're a medical cannabis patient, you might be allowed to grow more plants or have more lenient rules overall, but this often comes with mandatory registration or licensing. Patients usually must have a valid medical card, and their grows might be subject to inspections or inventory tracking. Recreational growers, meanwhile, might face tighter limits but don't have to go through paperwork or state health systems. Understanding which category your grow operation fits into ensures you follow the correct legal framework.

While the law might seem complex and sometimes overwhelming, there's a reason behind all these restrictions. Cannabis remains illegal at the federal level, which influences state lawmaking and enforcement. State legislators try to balance public safety, tax revenue, and social fairness, often tailoring laws to local attitudes about cannabis use. But the federal ban keeps things complicated, especially when it comes to transporting cannabis or selling it across state lines. For home growers, staying within state and local rules helps avoid entangling themselves in federal issues.

Many growers find it helpful to keep up with legal developments regularly. Cannabis laws are evolving rapidly as more states legalize and refine their regulations. What's allowed today might change next year or even within a few months. Signing up for newsletters from trustworthy cannabis legal organizations or joining local grower communities can provide timely information. Remaining proactive keeps you on the right side of the law and helps you adapt your growing plans accordingly.

Furthermore, maintaining good relationships with neighbors and your community plays a role in legal safety. Even if you follow every letter of the law, complaints about smells, lighting, or security might draw unwanted attention from local authorities. Taking steps to minimize odor through ventilation or carbon filters and ensuring your grow area is discreet can help prevent issues. Many growers find that mutual respect and open communication with nearby residents go a long way toward peaceful, uninterrupted cultivation.

When it comes to enforcement, penalties for breaking cannabis cultivation laws vary widely as well. Minor infractions, such as growing a few extra plants, could lead to fines or confiscation, while more serious violations might result in criminal charges or probation. Some states offer reduced penalties or opportunities to resolve charges quickly for first-time offenders. Knowing the specific consequences in your jurisdiction helps you weigh risks and make better-informed choices about your grow operation.

It's also worth noting that these laws don't just apply to the act of growing. Transporting cannabis from your grow site, sharing it with others, or selling it—even informally—can come with their own legal restrictions. Some states allow home cultivation strictly for personal use, prohibiting any sales or distribution. Others have clear rules separating personal growing from commercial licensing. Ignorance of these finer points can cause growers to unintentionally cross legal boundaries. If you want to eventually scale up, it's essential to understand

and respect the distinction between personal and commercial cultivation.

One handy tip is to document your compliance efforts. Keeping detailed records such as receipts for seeds, licenses, or registrations—and even photos of your grow setup—can serve as proof of legal compliance if you ever face scrutiny. While not all growers will need to produce such documentation, having it on hand offers peace of mind and can simplify matters if questions arise.

Lastly, consulting with a cannabis-knowledgeable attorney can be a wise investment, especially for those planning larger grows or those in states with particularly complex regulations. Legal counsel can clarify ambiguous areas, assist with paperwork, and help you anticipate potential pitfalls. While not every grower needs a lawyer, having access to expert advice provides a safety net that could save time, money, and stress in the long run.

Ultimately, mastering local and state cannabis laws is one of the most important foundations for a successful home grow. It shields you from trouble, respects your community, and allows you to focus on what matters most: nurturing healthy plants and producing quality cannabis. By doing your homework and keeping up with changing regulations, you build your grow operation on a solid, legal footing that supports sustainable and responsible cultivation.

Ethical and Responsible Growing for the Future

As cannabis cultivation continues to gain mainstream acceptance, it becomes increasingly important for growers to embrace ethical and responsible practices that support not only their plants but also the larger ecosystem and community. Growing cannabis sustainably isn't just about avoiding legal troubles or maximizing yields; it's about fostering a long-term mindset that respects the environment, honors local laws, and prioritizes social responsibility. This outlook ensures the industry's positive impact expands—not just now, but for years to come.

Ethical growing starts with an awareness of the broader consequences your growing choices have on nature. Whether you're cultivating a small home garden or running a sizable indoor operation, your decisions regarding water usage, energy consumption, waste management, and pesticide use ripple outward. Minimizing waste and embracing renewable resources can reduce your operation's carbon footprint, safeguarding natural habitats and conserving precious resources. At the same time, avoiding harmful chemicals protects beneficial insects and soil health, supporting a balanced ecosystem that benefits both your crop and the earth beneath it.

Being a responsible grower also means keeping a pulse on compliance with local and state regulations. Laws around cannabis cultivation often seek not just to manage supply but to ensure safety and community well-being. Following these rules builds trust between cultivators, consumers, and regulators alike. It also helps prevent negative outcomes such as overproduction, diversion into illegal markets, or neighborhood disputes. Staying informed about licensing requirements, plant limits, and reporting obligations keeps your grow legitimate, smooth, and worry-free.

Looking ahead, the future of cannabis growing hinges on collaboration and transparency. Sharing knowledge and practices within the community is essential for creating a culture of sustainability and ethics. Many growers find that openly exchanging tips on organic nutrients, pest management, and water-saving techniques elevates the entire industry's standards. This is especially true as new cultivators enter the scene, eager to learn but driven to avoid previous mistakes. By mentoring others and nurturing a supportive network, every responsible grower helps cultivate a healthier market and environment.

One challenge facing ethical growers is striking a balance between high-quality output and sustainable methods. High yields and potent buds typically demand more resources, such as intense lighting or tailored nutrient regimens. However, sustainable growers often innovate by integrating efficient technology and natural inputs instead of defaulting to heavy energy use or synthetic chemicals. For example, LED lighting systems reduce electricity consumption while delivering optimal light spectra for cannabis growth. Similarly, organic amendments improve soil health over time, promoting vigorous plants without polluting water sources or soil.

Another important aspect of responsibility lies in social equity and community engagement. Historically, cannabis prohibition disproportionately affected marginalized communities, so contemporary growers must consider how their practices can support fairness and healing. This means advocating for equitable policies, supporting local economies, and fostering inclusivity in all areas of cannabis culture. Some growers volunteer their time or donate a portion of their harvest to medical relief programs. Others actively participate in local initiatives that educate about safe consumption or destigmatize cannabis use. These efforts help repair past harms while strengthening the social fabric around the plant.

When it comes to environmental stewardship, simple habits can produce lasting benefits. Reducing water waste is critical, especially in regions prone to drought. Techniques like drip irrigation, rainwater harvesting, and collecting condensate from air filtration systems make water use more efficient and less burdensome on regional supplies. Additionally, composting plant waste rather than discarding it keeps organic matter cycling back into the soil instead of polluting landfills. Even using biodegradable pots and packaging aids in cutting down on plastics that threaten ecosystems worldwide.

Beyond environmental concerns, ethical growing also involves respecting neighbors and communities. Many growers have encountered challenges with odors, visibility, or noise, which can strain relationships and fuel stigma. Proactively addressing these issues—through carbon filtration, soundproofing, and discreet site planning—demonstrates respect and helps create a more positive perception of home cultivation. Responsible communication about your grow operation can promote understanding and reduce conflicts, which benefits everyone involved.

Looking forward, technological advancements offer exciting possibilities for making cannabis cultivation more sustainable and transparent. Smart automation systems can carefully monitor and adjust environmental factors to avoid wasteful energy or nutrient use. Data analytics enable growers to predict and prevent stress or disease, reducing the need for pesticides. Blockchain and seed-to-sale tracking, meanwhile, ensure accountability in production and distribution chains, protecting consumers and supporting legitimate businesses. Embracing such innovations equips growers with tools to uphold ethics without sacrificing efficiency or quality.

Ethical and responsible growing is ultimately about mindset as much as methods. It invites growers to think holistically and critically about their impact—from soil microbes to neighborhood perceptions—and to act with generosity, patience, and foresight. Your commitment shapes more than the plants in your garden; it influences an emerging culture where cannabis is grown with care for people and planet alike. For both newcomers and seasoned cultivators, embedding this philosophy early in the journey can set a standard that other growers will follow, making a meaningful difference across the industry.

In summary, cultivating cannabis ethically demands integrating sustainable environmental practices, respecting legal boundaries, and fostering social responsibility. It requires diligent planning, continuous learning, and active community involvement. Every grow operation, regardless of scale, plays a part in building a future where cannabis is not only high quality and accessible but also produced in a way that honors nature and benefits society. By adopting these principles today, you're investing in a legacy of ethical cultivation that will endure far beyond a single harvest.

Chapter 13
Selecting Cannabis Strains for Success

Choosing the right cannabis strain sets the foundation for a rewarding growing experience, blending your personal preferences with your cultivation goals. Whether you're after a strain with uplifting effects, medicinal benefits, or high yields, understanding the genetic background helps steer you toward plants that suit your climate, grow space, and patience level. Beginners often benefit from hardy, resilient strains that tolerate minor mistakes, while seasoned growers can experiment with more specialized genetics to chase unique flavors and potent effects. Strain selection isn't just about THC or CBD content; it's about balancing characteristics like growth time, plant size, and resistance to pests or mold to match your environment and lifestyle. By aligning your strain choice with these factors, you increase the chances of a successful harvest and enjoyable results that keep you motivated for future grows.

Understanding Strain Genetics and Effects

When it comes to choosing the right cannabis strain for your grow, understanding genetics is absolutely key. Strain genetics are like the blueprint that dictates how the plant will develop, how much THC or CBD it contains, its overall growth pattern, and even the kind of effects it delivers when consumed. Genetics shape everything from the plant's height and flowering time to its resistance against pests and diseases. Without a solid grasp of strain genetics, you might find yourself overwhelmed by the seemingly endless options available on the market.

Cannabis strains are typically categorized into three main types: indica, sativa, and hybrid. These categories stem from their genetic lineage and have long been associated with distinct physical traits and effects. While the classic explanation portrays indica strains as stocky and relaxing, and sativas as tall and energizing, the reality is much more complex. True to genetics, most strains you'll find today are hybrids, meaning they carry genetics from both indica and sativa ancestors. This mixture creates a spectrum of effects and growth characteristics rather than clear-cut categories.

What makes strain genetics so fascinating—and essential to understand—is how they influence the chemical makeup of the plant, especially cannabinoids and terpenes. Cannabinoids like THC and CBD interact with the human body's endocannabinoid system to produce a variety of effects, from pain relief to psychoactive highs. Terpenes, the fragrant oils found in cannabis, add another layer, affecting aroma, flavor, and sometimes even the nature of the high or relaxation a strain offers. Since these chemical components are genetically controlled, knowing the strain's lineage gives you insight into what to expect both in the garden and in your experience after consumption.

Different strains also respond uniquely to environmental factors. Genetics can determine whether a plant thrives indoors or outdoors, how it handles temperature swings, or how resistant it is to common pests and mold issues. For growers interested in maximizing yield and potency, selecting genetics that align with the growing environment is crucial. Even if you're a beginner, starting with robust genetics can prevent frustration and losses down the line.

Some strains are bred for specific traits beyond potency and yield. Medicinal growers, for example, often prioritize genetics with higher CBD content and lower THC to avoid strong psychoactive effects while still benefiting from therapeutic properties. Recreational growers tend to look for strains with unique terpene profiles or higher THC percentages. Understanding these genetics-driven goals helps you tailor your choices to what matters most, whether that's relaxation, creativity, or symptom relief.

One important aspect of genetics to note is stability. Some strains are stable, meaning they consistently produce similar plants generation after generation. Others—especially highly hybridized or newly created crosses—might show more variation within seeds. If consistency is a priority, opting for stable, well-established strains is wise. This stability also affects your growing efforts; plants that differ drastically in size or flowering time can complicate your cultivation workflow and require extra attention.

Even the physical appearance of the plants is genetically influenced. The leaf shape, the density of buds, coloration, and even resin production fall back on the strain's DNA. Sometimes you'll see phenotypes within a strain that look and act quite differently—even though they share the same name. These variations called "pheno hunting" in the grower community, can help you select the best-performing phenotype for your particular setup and preferences.

Taking time to research parent strains and their genetic backgrounds pays off in multiple ways. Knowing the origins of a strain often reveals important traits like ideal climate or humidity range, expected flowering time, and yield potential. It also helps set realistic expectations about the plant's behavior and any unique care requirements. This knowledge empowers you to anticipate challenges and adjust your grow environment before issues arise.

There's also a cultural and historical aspect wrapped up in strain genetics. Some strains carry rich legacies tied to specific regions—like landrace strains from Afghanistan, Colombia, or Thailand—that have evolved through natural selection and long cultivation histories. These landraces serve as the genetic foundation for many modern hybrids you're likely to encounter. Exploring and understanding these roots connects you to cannabis's broader story while providing clues about the plant's natural strengths and quirks.

It's easy to get caught up in numerical values when looking at strains—focusing solely on THC percentages, for example. However, genetics influence much more than just potency. The overall experience hinges on complex interactions between a plant's cannabinoids and terpenes. For instance, two strains might have similar THC levels but differ wildly in effects because their terpene profiles evoke different feelings like uplift, sedation, or focus.

In practice, this means your success in growing cannabis goes beyond picking the "strongest" strain on the shelf. Instead, look for genetics that fit your goals, environment, and tolerance. Beginners especially benefit from strains known for ease of growth and reliable performance. These tend to have forgiving genetics that withstand minor errors in watering or nutrient balance without crashing. Experienced growers might lean toward rarer or more challenging genetics to push their cultivation skills and achieve unique flavors or effects.

Choosing genetics that suit your lifestyle is just as essential as matching them to your grow conditions. The effects you want after harvest—whether relaxation, mental clarity, energy, or pain relief—stem from the underlying genetic canvas of the plant. By understanding how genetics inform these traits, you can grow with intention instead of guessing, making the entire process more rewarding.

Finally, never underestimate the role of breeder reputation and seed source quality when it comes to genetics. Even the most promising strain can underperform if the seed bank isn't trustworthy or the genetics are misrepresented. Investing in reputable suppliers who prioritize genetic stability and authenticity ensures you start your grow on the right foot.

Overall, mastering strain genetics is a game changer for any cannabis grower. It connects you closely to the plant's biology, your cultivation environment, and your personal needs. With this understanding, you'll not only improve your grow's success rate but also enjoy a richer, more nuanced relationship with cannabis—from seed to harvest to consumption.

Strain Recommendations for Beginners and Experts

Choosing the right cannabis strain is one of the most important decisions you'll make when setting up your grow. Whether you're stepping into this hobby for the first time or looking to refine an already experienced approach, picking strains that fit your skill level, environment, and goals will dramatically impact your success. While growers often get excited chasing exotic or high-THC strains, it's vital to match the strain's complexity to your cultivation experience and resources to avoid unnecessary frustration or loss.

For beginners, a solid starting point is picking strains that are forgiving and resilient. These tend to handle minor mistakes better and have simpler care requirements. Indicas or indica-dominant hybrids are often recommended because they usually have shorter flowering periods, sturdier branches, and more predictable growth patterns. Strains like *Blueberry*, *Northern Lights*, and *Granddaddy Purple* have earned their reputation as reliable starters because they show consistent results with less hands-on intervention.

Autoflowering strains also deserve a mention for novices. These varieties automatically switch from vegetative growth to flowering based on age rather than light cycles, making them easier to manage indoors or outdoors without complicated light schedules. Strains like *Auto Lemon Haze* or *Lowryder* strip away some of the technical layers that come with photoperiod plants, allowing new growers to stay focused on general plant health while learning the basics.

More advanced growers have a wider playground, thanks to their familiarity with cultivation variables.

They're comfortable juggling strain-specific quirks—like longer flowering times, higher nutrient demands, or sensitivity to environmental conditions—which opens doors to plenty of exotic or high-THC hybrids that can reward meticulous care with exceptional yields and unique effects.

For experts, you might want to hone in on strains that push your skills and offer distinct challenges, such as rare sativas known for their thin leaves and longer flowering periods. These tend to require precise humidity and temperature control, alongside rigorous pruning techniques. Varieties like *Durban Poison* or *Super Silver Haze* are classics in this category. They'll often test your ability to optimize ventilation and lighting but pay off with potent cerebral highs and impressive terpene profiles.

Hybrids offer some of the most exciting opportunities for all levels because they blend indica and sativa characteristics in various proportions. They provide a balance in growth habits and effects that can be tailored to your goals. If you want a bit of everything, choosing hybrids like *Girl Scout Cookies* or *Wedding Cake* can provide rich flavor, moderate flowering times, and mixed effects—offering both a sense of relaxation and uplift. These strains suit growers aiming to cultivate buds that appeal to a broad range of consumers or personal preferences.

Another crucial consideration when selecting strains is the plant's cannabinoid and terpene profiles. For many beginners, focusing solely on THC content can be overwhelming or even counterproductive. Some strains with very high THC percentages require careful handling because their potency can affect sensory sensitivity to lighting or humidity, and they might be more susceptible to nutrient imbalances or pest problems. Instead, opting for strains with balanced THC and CBD or even CBD-dominant options can make the cultivation process less stressful and yield more versatile uses.

For instance, CBD-rich strains like *Harlequin* or *ACDC* are known for their calming effects and often possess growth traits that appeal to both newcomers and seasoned growers. These strains might flower a bit longer but offer great resistance to mold and pests, especially important in high-humidity environments or less controlled outdoor grows. If your main goal includes medicinal use or gentler recreational effects, this path is worth exploring early on.

When recommending strains, it's impossible to ignore the importance of your local climate and grow environment. Some strains thrive outdoors under direct sun and fluctuating temperatures, while others may wilt without the stability indoor setups provide. Beginners might find it worthwhile to pick strains adapted to their region or ones broadly considered hardy in variable conditions. This reduces the learning curve tied to environmental stress factors and allows you to focus more on mastering cultivation basics.

Experienced growers, conversely, benefit from understanding how to select strains that either maximize yields in controlled indoor environments or complement the prevailing outdoor climate by flowering late or resisting pests endemic to the area. For example, Mediterranean or desert-region strains often have natural resilience to drought and heat, while northern or temperate strains may resist cooler temperatures and shorter summers better. Dialing in strain choice this way lays the foundation for growing success before the first seed even hits the soil.

Besides growth traits, anticipate the complexity of managing the flowering period when making your strain selection. Beginners generally fare better with strains that finish flowering in 8 to 9 weeks. These shorter cycles mean less time for pests to develop and fewer decisions around controlling humidity peaks and snipping overly vigorous branches. Longer flowering sativas, which can stretch past 12 weeks, might prove daunting in early cultivation efforts and increase the likelihood of mold or bud rot if not monitored carefully.

On the flip side, veteran growers usually welcome longer flowering schedules because they offer a chance to cultivate strains with exceptional flavor profiles and cannabinoids that synthesize best during extended maturation. Strains like *Amnesia Haze* or *Lamb's Bread* represent this category. They require patients but reward that care with buds rich in complex aromas and nuanced effects that are often prized for both recreational and therapeutic purposes.

It's wise for all growers to consider the end use of their harvest when choosing strains. Are you growing primarily for personal consumption, gifting, or perhaps small-scale sales within legal limits? This goal shapes whether you prioritize aroma, potency, yield, or ease of growth. Beginners often benefit from strains that deliver a balanced mix—reliable potency, pleasant flavor, and hearty structure—so that the learning experience is enjoyable and fosters enthusiasm for future grows.

For experts, tailoring strain selection toward niche markets or personal satisfaction becomes possible. Cultivators might look for rare landrace strains or crossbreeds that produce distinctive terpene profiles—unique smells and flavors that stand out in a crowded market or offer a one-of-a-kind sensory experience. Advanced cultivators also have the skills to manipulate environmental factors and training techniques that unlock the full potential of these more demanding strains.

Finally, don't overlook genetics as a foundation for success. Reliable seed banks and breeders provide detailed strain descriptions that go beyond THC levels, illustrating growth habits, resistance traits, and effects. Beginners should pick seeds from reputable sources that guarantee stable genetics to avoid surprises such as hermaphroditism or unpredictable growth patterns. Experts may experiment with preserving heirloom cultivars or breeding their own hybrids once they're confident in maintaining healthy parent plants.

In summary, strain selection starts with understanding personal needs, environment, and experience. For beginners, look for hardy, short-flowering indicas or autoflowers to build confidence and skills. Intermediate growers can explore hybrid varieties balancing multiple traits, while advanced cultivators can dive into rare sativas and specialized genetics that challenge their precision and creativity. No matter your level, the right strain is a vital first step that sets the entire growing journey on the path to success.

Chapter 14
Building an Ideal Indoor Grow Room

Creating the perfect indoor grow room sets the foundation for a thriving cannabis garden, blending thoughtful planning with practical execution to shape an environment where your plants can truly flourish. From choosing a space that allows for adequate room to move and tend to your plants, to ensuring precise control over temperature, humidity, and airflow, every detail matters when building a setup that promotes healthy growth. Effective placement of lighting systems tailored to the needs of your cannabis strains pairs with ventilation strategies that keep air fresh and prevent mold or pests, making the difference between mediocre and exceptional yields. By envisioning your grow room as a dynamic ecosystem that demands balance and attention, you position yourself to cultivate resilient plants with vibrant buds, all within the comfort and privacy of your own space.

Room Setup and Environmental Control

Setting up an ideal indoor grow room goes far beyond just picking the right lights or pots. The environment you create inside that space will dictate how well your cannabis plants thrive. In fact, controlling temperature, humidity, airflow, and cleanliness can be just as crucial as the genetics of your plants. If these factors aren't dialed in properly, you could end up with stunted growth, mold issues, or poor yields—even if everything else is perfect.

Start by choosing an appropriate space for your grow room. It should be a room you can dedicate solely to your cannabis cultivation without frequent interruptions. Privacy and security are important, but so is the room's natural insulation. Closets, spare bedrooms, or small basements often make excellent grow rooms because they can be easily modified to maintain a stable environment. Avoid spots prone to heavy temperature swings or drafts, like near exterior doors or windows that don't seal tightly.

Once you've selected your space, think about how you'll control temperature. Cannabis plants generally prefer temperatures between 70 and 85 degrees Fahrenheit during their light cycles, dipping slightly lower during the dark periods. Installing a reliable thermostat-controlled heater or air conditioner can keep your grow room within this ideal range. Temperature fluctuations, especially extreme highs or lows, stress plants and can slow development or even cause damage. Using a space with good insulation helps reduce the energy needed to keep temperatures stable.

Humidity control is equally important. During the vegetative stage, cannabis favors relative humidity levels around 40 to 70 percent, but this needs to drop to 40 to 50 percent during flowering to avoid mold and bud rot. Without a dehumidifier or humidifier, it's tough to maintain those precise levels. If you start noticing condensation on leaves or walls, it's your cue to add a dehumidifier. Conversely, very dry air can cause problems too, so a humidifier might be necessary in arid climates or heated rooms. Keep a reliable hygrometer handy to constantly monitor these levels.

Air circulation and ventilation deserve special attention, though they're topics explored further later on. In this section, the focus is on the basics of setting up your room's airflow pathways. Proper ventilation isn't just about freshness—it helps regulate temperature and humidity, supplies carbon dioxide for photosynthesis, and strengthens plant stems by simulating natural wind. Install oscillating fans or clip fans strategically to promote steady airflow without causing direct blasts on your plants, since that might stress them. Make sure fresh air can enter, ideally from cooler, filtered sources, and stale air exhausts out efficiently.

Sanitation is often overlooked but lays the foundation for a healthy grow environment. Before setting up, clean the entire grow space thoroughly. Wipe down walls, floors, and shelves with non-toxic disinfectants safe for indoor plants. Avoid bringing outside dirt or pests inside; change clothes and shoes, or use clean covers when working in the space. Once your grow room is in operation, regular cleaning routines minimize mold spores, dust, and insect pest buildup, keeping your plants safe and vigorous.

Light reflections inside the grow room affect how evenly your plants receive light. Painting walls with flat white or using specialized reflective materials can increase light efficiency, bouncing photons back onto the canopy instead of letting them get absorbed by dark walls or floors. This simple tweak helps your plants soak up more usable light without needing to crank up electricity consumption. Just remember, avoid shiny surfaces that create hotspots, as these can actually harm delicate leaves.

Consider the layout of your grow space carefully. Arrange pots or containers so each plant gets an equal share of light and airflow. Crowding plants too close limits their access to carbon dioxide and can trap excess moisture, creating hotspots for mold. Conversely, spreading plants too far apart wastes available grow room space and your lighting setup. Finding that sweet spot depends on your choice of strain, growth style, and lighting type, but a well-organized floor plan makes maintenance and harvesting easier too.

Environmental control also involves managing electrical setups responsibly. Indoor grow rooms require multiple power-hungry pieces of equipment—lights, fans, humidifiers, and more—which means you should avoid daisy-chaining too many devices on a single outlet. Use surge protectors, circuit breakers, and possibly consult an electrician to ensure your wiring is safe and adequate for the load. Nothing puts a damper on your grow like blown fuses or worse, fire hazards.

Another element to keep in mind is the room's sealability. You want a space that can be sealed tightly to better control air exchanges and block smells, but not so airtight that airflow suffers. Sealing windows and gaps is crucial for smell management and maintaining stable environmental conditions. Using carbon filters in exhaust systems really helps keep odors in check, especially where discretion is an issue. A solidly sealed room also reduces contamination risks from pests or airborne spores.

Technology makes environmental control more accessible than ever. Digital controllers can automate routines that manage temperature, humidity, and even lighting schedules precisely. These tools free you from constant monitoring and help avoid human errors. Setting alarms on your environmental devices ensures you catch issues early, whether it's a spike in temperature or a malfunctioning fan. Of course, nothing replaces good old-fashioned observation—regularly inspect your plants and room for signs of stress or equipment failure.

While this section covers the fundamental framework of room setup and environmental control, it forms the backbone for everything discussed in later sections—like lighting selection or ventilation strategies. If you master creating a stable and healthy environment first, your cannabis plants will thank you with lush growth and impressive yields. The initial effort to design and control these factors pays off in peace of mind during your grow cycles and ultimately, a successful harvest.

In essence, building your grow room is like setting the stage for a play; the plants are the actors and environmental controls the director. The better your room replicates the ideal climate cannabis plants crave, the easier your job becomes. So invest the time and attention now to get your room's setup right, and you'll pave a smooth path toward growing high-quality cannabis at home.

Choosing Lighting Systems to Maximize Growth

Lighting is one of the most critical elements when it comes to building an ideal indoor grow room for cannabis cultivation. Without the right type and intensity of light, your plants simply won't reach their full potential. Choosing the proper lighting system can feel overwhelming at first, especially with so many options on the market, but understanding the basics will help you make an informed decision that fits your space, budget, and goals.

At its core, cannabis plants rely on light as their energy source for photosynthesis. Indoor growers must replicate the sun's natural light spectrum and intensity since plants won't get much help from the environment like in an outdoor garden. The quality, spectrum, and duration of the light you provide directly impact growth rates, branching, bud production, and overall health. A well-chosen lighting system not only boosts yields but also improves resin development, contributing to better potency and aroma.

One important factor to consider is the growth stage of your plants. During the vegetative phase, they thrive under higher intensities of blue light that encourage sturdy structure and healthy leaf development. When transitioning to flowering, plants benefit from red and orange wavelengths that stimulate bud formation and maturation. Some lighting setups allow you to adjust the spectrum throughout these phases, optimizing energy use and plant response. This adaptability can significantly improve crop quality with relatively little extra effort.

Traditional High-Intensity Discharge (HID) lights, including Metal Halide (MH) and High-Pressure Sodium (HPS) bulbs, have long been the go-to choices for indoor cannabis growing. MH lights emit a bluer light spectrum suitable for vegetative growth, while HPS produce red and orange hues more conducive to flowering. These lamps have proven effectiveness and robust light intensity, making them reliable in many grow rooms. However, they also produce significant heat, which demands good ventilation and climate control to avoid stressing your plants.

In contrast, Light Emitting Diode (LED) technology has become increasingly popular among growers looking for energy efficiency and customizable light spectra. Modern LED grow lights offer full-spectrum output, often tailored specifically for cannabis plants, along with lower electricity consumption and reduced heat generation. This means you can maintain optimal temperature conditions with less need for bulky ventilation systems. LEDs tend to last longer than traditional bulbs, making them cost-effective over time despite a higher initial investment.

Another emerging option is Ceramic Metal Halide (CMH) or Light Emitting Ceramic (LEC) lights, which combine some advantages of HID and LED styles. CMH lamps emit a broad spectrum of light, including ultraviolet (UV) wavelengths that may enhance trichome production and plant defense. They run somewhat cooler than traditional HPS systems and generally boast longer lifespans. Though CMH fixtures often come with a steeper price tag, many growers find their quality-to-cost ratio attractive, particularly for mid-sized to large setups.

A vital consideration when choosing any lighting system is the coverage area relative to the size of your grow space. Too little light means weak, leggy plants with subpar yields, while too much intensity can burn leaves and waste power. Manufacturers provide guidelines indicating how many square feet a particular fixture can effectively cover. For most home growers, it's better to use multiple smaller units spaced evenly rather than one oversized light to ensure uniformity and avoid hotspots or shaded zones.

Reflectivity within the grow room also impacts how efficiently your lighting performs. Surfaces like Mylar, white paint, or reflective grow tents help bounce light back onto your plants, increasing exposure without cranking up wattage. This simple adjustment can make a noticeable difference in growth without additional expenses. When planning your room setup, think about how your chosen lighting system interacts with wall materials and fixture placement to maximize effective light delivery.

Managing light cycles is another crucial part of maximizing cannabis growth. During vegetative growth, plants often need 18 to 24 hours of light each day, depending on the strain. When it's time to flower, growers typically switch to a 12/12 light/dark schedule to trigger bud development. Choosing a lighting system that allows easy scheduling and reliable operation will save you headaches. Some LED models come with integrated timers or smart controls that let you adjust spectral output and timing via apps, which can be extremely handy for hands-off management.

Heat output and energy consumption shouldn't be overlooked during your decision-making process. HID systems tend to produce more heat, which means investing in good ventilation and cooling solutions to maintain stable temperatures between 70 and 85 degrees Fahrenheit. Excessive heat can stunt growth or increase moisture stress, making your plants vulnerable to diseases. LEDs, meanwhile, run cooler and often drastically lower electric bills, an advantage many growers appreciate—especially for continuous or large-scale operations.

Certain growers also incorporate supplemental lighting when extending day length or boosting intensity in dense canopies. Side lighting or adjustable fixtures positioned within the plant canopy can increase light penetration to lower branches, resulting in more even growth and higher overall yields. This setup is more common among experienced cultivators who understand canopy management but is worth mentioning as it speaks to the versatility and creativity you can apply in lighting your grow room.

In terms of cost, your budget will largely dictate which lighting systems are viable. HID setups tend to have lower upfront costs, but replacement bulbs and higher energy use add expenses over time. LED systems may require more initial spending, but their longevity and efficiency often lead to savings in the long run. Weighing those costs against expected yields and growth quality will help you pick a system that balances performance and affordability.

Ultimately, the best lighting system for maximizing growth depends on your specific space, experience level, and cultivation goals. Whether you opt for traditional HID lamps, efficient LEDs, or versatile CMH fixtures, understanding how each type influences your plants' life cycle is essential. Pay close attention to how light intensity, spectrum, coverage, and heat output interact within your grow room environment. When done right, the perfect lighting setup becomes the backbone of a successful indoor cannabis garden.

Ventilation and Airflow for Healthy Plants

Ventilation is often overlooked by beginners but plays a crucial role in building an ideal indoor grow room. Proper airflow isn't just about keeping the room from feeling stale—it directly impacts the health and vigor of your cannabis plants throughout their lifecycle. Without adequate ventilation, you risk creating stagnant, humid conditions that can lead to mold, pests, and weak stems. On the flip side, well-managed airflow encourages strong growth, efficient gas exchange, and temperature control, all of which are vital for maximizing yield and resin production.

Think of your grow room as a living ecosystem, where air acts like the bloodstream carrying oxygen in and carbon dioxide out. Cannabis plants breathe much like we do—they consume carbon dioxide during photosynthesis and release oxygen, especially in well-lit environments. If the air sits still around the leaves for too long, plants don't get the fresh CO2 they need, which slows down photosynthesis and growth. Good ventilation constantly replaces old air with fresh air rich in carbon dioxide, creating an environment where your plants can breathe freely and grow robustly.

Airflow also influences temperature and humidity, two critical environmental factors in cannabis cultivation. During the flowering stage alone, plants generate a considerable amount of heat and moisture, which can quickly build up in a confined space. Without sufficient air movement, these conditions create a perfect breeding ground for powdery mildew, bud rot, and other fungal problems that can devastate your crop. Proper ventilation systems help remove excess heat and moisture, maintaining balanced conditions and lessening the risk of diseases.

When setting up ventilation, it helps to think in terms of both air exchange and internal airflow. Air exchange refers to bringing fresh air in and pushing stale air out of the grow space. This is usually done with intake and exhaust fans. Intake fans pull fresh air from outside the room or grow tent, while exhaust fans expel hot, humid air to the outside. Strategically placing these fans—often with the intake fan near the bottom and the exhaust fan near the top—leverages natural convection, as warm air rises and can be pulled out more efficiently.

Internal airflow, meanwhile, is about circulating air within the room to prevent pockets of still air around your plants. Oscillating fans, clip fans, or circulating fans placed inside the grow space keep the air moving gently across all parts of the plants. This steady breeze simulates natural outdoor conditions, strengthening stems and promoting transpiration, which is the plant's natural process of releasing water vapor. A light, consistent airflow also helps plants regulate their temperature and prevents the formation of microclimates where humidity and temperature might fluctuate wildly.

Choosing the right fans and ventilation equipment depends on the size of your grow room and the intensity of your grow lights. Powerful lighting generates a lot of heat, so heavier airflow might be necessary to keep temperatures in check. A common guideline is to calculate how many times per minute you want your entire volume of air replaced—usually between 1 and 3 exchanges per minute. For example, a 4-foot by 4-foot tent with an 8-foot height holds about 128 cubic feet of air, so your exhaust fan should be capable of moving roughly 128 to 384 cubic feet per minute (CFM) of air.

Carbon filters often get incorporated into ventilation systems, particularly when odor control is a concern during the flowering phase. These filters attach to the exhaust fan and use activated carbon to neutralize strong cannabis smells before the air leaves the grow room. While not part of airflow itself, they're critical to maintaining discretion and preventing odor from becoming an issue, especially in shared living spaces or places with close neighbors.

Aside from fans and filters, it's smart to consider the direction of airflow in relation to how you arrange your plants. Air entering should flow over the canopy but not be so strong as to physically stress or damage the leaves. Too much wind can cause leaf fluttering, which might slow growth or cause mechanical stress, while too little won't provide adequate circulation. Adjust fan speeds using controllers or variable speed fans to find the perfect balance.

Humidity management is closely tied to ventilation as well. Young seedlings and clones thrive in higher humidity—usually between 65% and 70%—but mature flowering plants prefer much lower humidity, often around 40% to 50%. As your plants move through growth stages, adjusting ventilation rates helps regulate these changes. Higher airflow removes moisture faster, helping to drop humidity levels during flowering and reducing the risk of mold on dense buds.

Many growers use timers or environmental monitors in combination with ventilation equipment to automate air exchange based on temperature and humidity readings. This ensures conditions remain optimal even when you're not around to manually adjust settings. Simple hygrometers or smart sensors can alert you if the environment shifts outside preferred thresholds, prompting a fan speed adjustment or turning on additional ventilation.

Another factor worth considering is the introduction of fresh air and where it's drawn from. Ideally, intakes should bring in fresh, clean air from outside your grow room or even your home's ventilation system, avoiding air that's already hot or humid. Some growers use passive intakes where the fan creates negative pressure inside the tent, gently drawing air in through small intake vents without an active intake fan. This method saves energy and reduces noise but depends heavily on creating an airtight exhaust system.

Sound management also goes hand-in-hand with ventilation. Fans can generate a noticeable hum or vibration, especially in small indoor setups. Using ducting, vibration pads, or noise-insulating materials around fans can help keep your grow environment quieter. This isn't just a comfort issue; excessive noise can sometimes attract unwanted attention or disrupt your peace of mind.

Successful ventilation impacts plant health beyond just creating comfortable air conditions. It encourages stronger structural development as stems respond positively to airflow, thickening and becoming better equipped to support heavy buds. Infused terpenes and cannabinoids also develop fully in well-ventilated rooms because plants aren't stressed by excessive heat or humidity.

Finally, ventilation isn't a set-it-and-forget-it component. It demands regular maintenance: cleaning fans, checking ducting for blockages, and ensuring filters don't clog over time. Neglecting these details can quickly reduce airflow efficiency and undermine your efforts. Keeping ventilation equipment in top condition is a small investment that pays huge dividends in plant performance and overall grow success.

In summary, adequate ventilation and proper airflow form the backbone of a thriving indoor cannabis grow. They're the invisible forces that keep your plants breathing, dry, and healthy, safeguarding against common pitfalls like mold, pests, and heat stress. By prioritizing these elements early, you lay down a solid foundation that will help your cannabis grow from seedlings into dense, resinous colas worth the effort.

Chapter 15
Outdoor Growing Fundamentals

Growing cannabis outdoors taps into nature's full potential, offering plants access to natural sunlight, fresh air, and ample space to thrive, but it also demands careful preparation and ongoing attention to the environment you're working with. Choosing the right spot means understanding your local climate, soil quality, and exposure to sunlight—elements that set the stage for a healthy, robust crop. Seasonal changes play a big role outdoors, so knowing when to plant and how to protect your garden from unpredictable weather or pests will keep your plants strong from seedling to harvest. Unlike indoor growing, you can't control every variable with a switch or a dial, but with smart planning and an eye for your surroundings, outdoor cultivation can yield amazing results that connect you directly to the natural rhythm your plants crave.

Preparing Your Outdoor Grow Site

Choosing the right outdoor grow site is the foundation of a successful cannabis cultivation. You could have the best seeds and perfect growing know-how, but if your location isn't up to par, your crop will struggle. When scouting for a spot, think about sunlight first. Cannabis plants need ample direct sunlight—ideally 6 to 8 hours a day—to produce dense, potent buds. If your plot is shaded by trees or buildings for much of the day, yields will likely suffer.

Another vital factor is the soil quality at your chosen site. Cannabis thrives in well-draining, moderately fertile soil with good organic content. Heavy clay or overly sandy soil can cause root issues or prevent your plants from accessing enough nutrition. You'll want to test the soil composition and pH before planting. A pH between 6.0 and 7.0 works best. Too acidic or alkaline soil can lock out nutrients, even if they're plentiful.

Drainage and water availability go hand in hand with soil considerations. Stagnant water around roots invites problems like root rot and mold, so ensure your spot doesn't hold water after a rain. On the flip side, having easy access to a clean water source will make watering routines much easier. If you're miles from a faucet or well, it might be worth rethinking the site or preparing for additional infrastructure to meet your hydration needs.

Security is often overlooked but absolutely critical. Outdoor grows can be vulnerable to theft or unwanted attention, especially for cannabis. You want a location that's discreet but also accessible enough for regular care and monitoring. Some growers hide their crops behind natural barriers like dense shrubs or tall grass, while others use fencing and even motion-activated lights to protect their investment.

Prepare your site by clearing away debris, rocks, and any plants that might compete with your cannabis. If you're setting up in a new area, consider the presence of local wildlife. Deer, rabbits, and other critters can decimate young plants quickly, so adding fencing or repellents before planting pays off. Even if you haven't seen pests around, it's better to be proactive.

Topography plays a subtle but important role too. Flat land often allows easier water distribution and maintenance, but gentle slopes can offer better drainage. Steep angles, on the other hand, might cause erosion and wash away your soil nutrients. Observe how the land behaves after a rainfall to get clues about its suitability.

Climate patterns must also be factored into your site preparation strategy. While you can't control the weather, choosing a microclimate that protects your plants from extreme winds or sudden temperature swings can make a difference. Areas near bodies of water tend to have more moderate temperatures. Likewise, avoid low-lying, frost-prone spots that could cause early damage in sensitive growth stages.

When it comes to setting up physical support, consider staking or trellising frameworks before your plants get too big. Outdoor cannabis can become top-heavy in late flowering, especially indicas or hybrids with dense buds. Installing supports early prevents damage from wind gusts or heavy colas pulling branches down. You can use natural materials like bamboo poles or durable garden stakes combined with soft ties to avoid cutting into stems.

Cultivating a protective barrier against pests and environmental stress will boost your plants' chances of thriving. Many growers use natural mulch layers around the base of plants to retain soil moisture, regulate temperature, and discourage weed growth. Organic mulches, such as straw or shredded leaves, also break down nutrients slowly, enriching the soil. Just ensure mulch doesn't touch the stems directly, as that can invite rot.

Outdoor growers often have to anticipate seasonal challenges, so maintaining flexibility in your site plans helps. For example, you might want to build temporary shade structures for harsh midday sun or windbreaks to shelter against storms. While detailed weather management falls into a different topic, setting aside space and resources for these adjustments during site preparation smooths your path forward during the growing season.

Finally, don't forget about airflow. Good ventilation around your cannabis plants reduces the risk of mold and mildew decimating your harvest. When clearing your site, trim back overly dense vegetation nearby to allow breezes to circulate freely. Natural wind helps strengthen stalks and washes away excess humidity, which is crucial in outdoor crop health.

Taking these steps upfront in preparing your outdoor grow site lays the groundwork for a high-quality cannabis harvest. A well-chosen, prepped location supports healthy root development, strong plants, and better resistance to environmental stressors. You'll start the season confident that your plants have everything they need to flourish. From here, it's all about consistent care, attentive monitoring, and adapting as your garden grows.

Seasonal Considerations for Outdoor Cultivation

Growing cannabis outdoors brings a unique set of rewards and challenges, many of which hinge on the seasons. Unlike indoor growing, where conditions can be tightly controlled, outdoor cultivation relies heavily on nature's schedule. Understanding the seasonal rhythms and planning accordingly is crucial for a successful outdoor grow. The interplay of sunlight, temperature, rainfall, and pests changes as the year progresses, and your cannabis plants will respond to these shifts. Anticipating these variations can make the difference between an abundant harvest and a disappointing yield.

The starting point for any outdoor grow is timing your planting to match your local climate. Cannabis thrives in long, warm days loaded with sunlight, so knowing when the frost dates hit in your region is essential. Planting too early risks cold damage or slow growth, while planting too late can force your plants into flowering prematurely or not reaching full maturity. This is especially true in areas with short growing seasons. Beginners often underestimate how critical this timing is; pushing seeds into the ground before conditions are stable can compromise plant vigor from the get-go.

Spring is generally the time when outdoor growers kick off their grows. Early spring offers gradually increasing daylight hours, which stimulates vegetative growth. However, spring weather can be unpredictable, swinging from chilly nights to sudden rains. Frost can still occur after seedlings emerge, so protection methods like cloches, row covers, or even greenhouses can help shield young plants in this vulnerable phase. For growers at higher elevations or northern latitudes, starting your plants indoors or in a controlled environment before transplanting outdoors can bridge this gap effectively.

As summer approaches, cannabis plants typically enter their peak vegetative phase, bolstered by long, sunny days and generally warm temperatures. Outdoor growers should take advantage of this period to provide ample space and nutrients for explosive plant growth. It's also the time when watering becomes a more frequent task since increased heat and sunaccelerate soil moisture evaporation. While summer brings growth opportunities, it also means being vigilant about heat stress and potential pest invasions, both of which tend to ramp up as temperatures climb.

Light length plays a pivotal role in outdoor cannabis cultivation, especially as the seasons change. Cannabis is photoperiod-sensitive, which means the plant's flowering cycle initiates when the nights grow longer past a certain threshold. For most outdoor strains, this happens as summer fades into fall. Pay attention to local daylight trends so you can anticipate when your plants will naturally switch from vegetative growth to flowering. This timing influences everything from nutrient adjustments to pest management strategies, as flowering plants have different needs than vegetative ones.

Approaching fall brings cooler temperatures and shorter days, heralding the flowering stage outdoors. This phase demands extra care because the environmental conditions become less predictable. Early fall rains can increase humidity, which raises the risk of mold and bud rot—a serious threat for dense cannabis flowers. Adequate airflow around and within the canopy becomes essential, so strategic pruning and plant spacing are great preventative steps. Choosing strains that mature quickly or have some resistance to moisture-related problems can also pay dividends in wetter fall climates.

Fall is also when growers must start preparing for the impending harvest. Since outdoor crops are bound by the natural cycle, you can't delay harvest indefinitely without risking overripe or spoiled buds. The right harvest window ensures optimal potency and flavor, but weather can interfere—especially if autumn storms become severe. Keeping a close eye on your plants' trichomes and pistils will help you decide the best moment to chop, even if the forecast is less than ideal. Sometimes, it's better to harvest a bit early rather than risk losing your entire crop to weather damage.

Winter generally marks the end of the outdoor growing season, and for many regions, this means the plants will have completed their life cycle. After harvest, many growers use this downtime to prepare for the next season, by amending soil, cleaning tools, and planning their next grow. However, in milder climates, some gardeners experiment with extending the outdoor season by using protective structures or selecting hardy autoflowering strains that can tolerate cooler temperatures. These strategies can help squeeze out an extra harvest or two, but they require a clear understanding of your local climate's winter patterns.

Seasonal pests and diseases follow a similar timeline, often emerging when conditions become favorable in particular parts of the year. For example, aphids and spider mites like warmer months but can retreat when conditions dry out or cool down. Powdery mildew and bud rot tend to spike during humid, damp periods typical of late summer and fall. Seasonally adjusting your pest management approach helps minimize infestations, protecting your plants without excessive chemical use. Incorporating integrated pest management (IPM) techniques tailored to the seasons will keep your grow both safer and more sustainable.

Rainfall is another seasonal factor outdoor growers can't afford to ignore. Wet conditions during critical growth phases can wash away nutrients, compact soil, and foster fungal issues. In regions with heavy rainy seasons, raised beds or well-draining soil mixes are beneficial to prevent waterlogged roots. Conversely, in drier climates, preparing for extended dry spells with efficient irrigation or mulching can ensure consistent plant hydration. Understanding the moisture patterns of your locale throughout the seasons helps in crafting a watering plan that complements natural rainfall variations.

Temperature swings, especially between day and night, gain prominence as the seasons transition. Cannabis plants generally prefer warm days and cooler nights, which can enhance terpene production and improve overall bud quality. However, extreme temperature drops or heat waves can stress plants severely. In spring and fall, nighttime temperatures dipping below 50°F (10°C) might slow growth or cause leaf damage. Utilizing thermal covers during cold spells or choosing planting spots with some thermal mass from rocks or buildings can moderate these swings.

Many outdoor growers find it valuable to track local seasonal changes throughout the year. Maintaining a grow journal with notes on weather, pest activity, and plant response over multiple seasons provides an invaluable reference. Patterns often emerge that can guide future planting and care decisions. You begin to anticipate when to start seedlings, when to ramp up watering, and when to be ready for pest invasions. This kind of seasonal awareness transforms outdoor cultivation from guesswork into a more predictable, manageable process.

It's worth noting that regional climate variations can be dramatic, even within the same country. Coastal areas, deserts, mountains, and plains each have distinct seasonal cues and challenges. For example, a grower in the Pacific Northwest might contend with cool, wet springs, a short summer, and early autumn rains, while someone in the Southwest faces intense heat and dryness during summer months. Tailoring your seasonal plan to these local realities, rather than relying on general rules, boosts your odds of success.

Lastly, growers often find that experimenting with different strains suited to their particular seasonal windows increases their chances of a thriving outdoor crop. Some varieties are bred to be fast finishers, perfect for short growing seasons. Others excel with longer, warmer summers. Even subtle differences in flowering time can mean the difference between harvesting before a killing frost or losing your plants to the cold. Looking beyond yield, consider how your chosen strain's performance aligns with your seasonal growing environment.

Mastering seasonal considerations for outdoor cannabis cultivation means embracing nature's clock while applying your own knowledge and adaptability. There's a dance between respecting the environment and pushing the limits of growth that many cultivators find deeply rewarding. Each passing season becomes a lesson in observation, adjustment, and patience—qualities that elevate your skills as a home grower and bring you closer to that perfect, sun-kissed harvest.

Protection From Weather and Pests Outdoors

Growing cannabis outdoors comes with the rewarding challenge of working with nature, but it also means your plants are exposed to a wide range of weather conditions and pesky invaders. Giving your garden the right kind of protection can make a huge difference in the health of your crop and the quality of your buds. It's not just about shielding plants from the obvious threats like storms or bugs; it's also about creating an environment that allows them to thrive despite these hurdles.

Weather is unpredictable, and outdoor growers need to be ready for heat waves, unexpected cold snaps, heavy rain, and strong winds. Each of these conditions can stress your plants, stunt growth, or even kill them if not properly managed. Starting with a good understanding of your local climate and seasonal patterns will help you plan the best time to plant and harvest. For example, planting too early in the season can expose young plants to frost and cold damage, while leaving plants in the late season too long invites the risk of mold from excess moisture.

One of the simplest yet most effective ways to shield your plants from harsh weather is through strategic site selection. Choosing a location with natural windbreaks, like a hedgerow or a row of trees, can reduce strong winds that might otherwise snap stems or uproot plants. If natural barriers aren't available, consider installing screens or fences designed to block gusts without completely blocking airflow, which is essential for preventing fungal diseases.

When it comes to protecting plants from heavy rain, drainage is key. Cannabis hates waterlogged roots, which can lead to root rot and other fungal infections. Raised beds or well-draining soil mixes help water move away from roots quickly. Additionally, covering your plants with temporary plastic tunnels or row covers during heavy rains can keep excess moisture off the buds and leaves, helping prevent mold while allowing light to pass through. These covers should be removed promptly once the storm passes to avoid overheating.

Temperature swings can be another challenge. Unexpected cold nights or heatwaves can stress plants, causing nutrient uptake problems or slowed growth. In colder climates, using cloches, cold frames, or frost blankets can protect young plants during chilly nights. For extreme heat, providing some afternoon shade with shade cloth can reduce heat stress and prevent leaves from getting scorched. It's a balancing act, as your plants still need plenty of sunlight, but avoiding the most intense midday rays often helps maintain healthy growth.

Now, on the topic of pests—nature provides plenty of common enemies that love to feast on cannabis. Aphids, spider mites, caterpillars, and thrips are just a few of the usual suspects. If left unchecked, these insects can severely damage your plants by sucking sap, munching leaves, or spreading disease. Prevention is always easier than treatment, so establishing a strong defense early on is crucial.

Physical barriers are an excellent first line of defense. Insect netting can keep flying pests out, while collars around stems can stop crawling insects. This method has the advantage of avoiding chemical sprays, which might harm beneficial insects or leave unwanted residues. Companion planting also works well—growing plants like marigolds, basil, or nasturtiums alongside cannabis can repel pests or attract predators that eat harmful bugs.

Encouraging beneficial insects is another natural strategy that pays off. Ladybugs, lacewings, and predatory wasps prey on common pests, helping keep their populations under control. Creating a diverse garden environment with flowering plants to nourish these helpful allies ensures they stick around. Remember, a balanced ecosystem is the best way to maintain plant health without having to resort to harsh chemicals.

When pest problems become serious, natural remedies like neem oil, insecticidal soaps, or diatomaceous earth offer effective options. These substances disrupt pest biology but are generally safe for your plants and the environment when applied correctly. However, always test any treatment on a small part of your plant first and avoid spraying during the hottest part of the day to prevent leaf burn.

In addition to insect pests, outdoor cannabis is vulnerable to larger animals such as deer, rabbits, and rodents. These critters will nibble on leaves and buds if they get the chance. Fencing is the most straightforward protection here. A sturdy wire mesh fence, at least six feet tall, can deter deer, while smaller mesh at the base prevents rabbits and rodents from burrowing under. For extra security, motion-activated lights or sprinklers can startle nocturnal visitors and keep them away.

Mildew and mold, especially powdery mildew and bud rot, pose constant threats in humid environments or during rainy seasons. These fungal diseases thrive on wet, stagnant air around densely packed foliage. To reduce the risk, keep your plants well-spaced to allow airflow, prune lower branches where moisture tends to settle, and harvest promptly once buds mature. Removing infected parts immediately and sanitizing tools helps stop spores from spreading throughout your garden.

All these protection strategies come together to create a resilient outdoor grow environment. Protection is not about completely isolating your plants from the weather or pests—after all, cannabis is hardy and evolved outdoors—but about managing these factors in a way that keeps your crop healthy and productive. By anticipating challenges and responding quickly, you'll avoid many common pitfalls that sabotage outdoor grows.

Finally, patience and observation are key. Spending time in your garden regularly to check for signs of weather damage or pest invasion means you'll catch problems early before they spiral out of control. Keeping a grow journal with notes on weather patterns and pest activity can help you fine-tune your protective measures season by season. Outdoor cannabis cultivation is a dynamic journey. With proper planning and care, your efforts will pay off with luscious, potent buds shaped by the very environment you nurture.

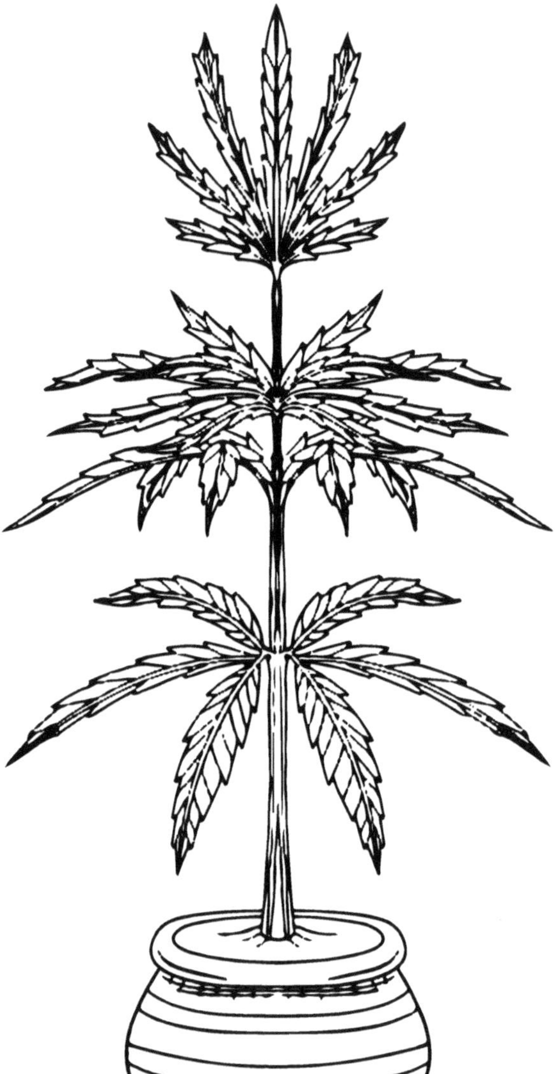

Chapter 16
Nutrient Management Strategies

Getting nutrient management right is crucial for growing healthy cannabis plants that deliver top-notch buds, and it's about more than just pouring in fertilizers. It's important to understand how different nutrients work together and when your plants need them most, adjusting feeding schedules as they move through their life cycle. Balancing macronutrients like nitrogen, phosphorus, and potassium with the essential micronutrients supports strong growth without risking nutrient burn or deficiencies. Choosing between organic and synthetic options often comes down to your growing style and goals—each has its benefits and challenges. Ultimately, fine-tuning your approach to feeding builds a solid foundation, helping your crop thrive from seedling to harvest without wasting resources or jeopardizing quality.

Macronutrients and Micronutrients Explained

When it comes to growing cannabis, nutrients are the foundation of healthy, vigorous plants. Whether you're just starting out or have been cultivating for years, understanding the difference between macronutrients and micronutrients is crucial. Both play distinct yet complementary roles in plant development, and by grasping these basics, you can avoid common mistakes that stunt growth or reduce yield and potency.

Macronutrients are the primary building blocks cannabis plants need in larger amounts. They include nitrogen (N), phosphorus (P), and potassium (K), often referred to as N-P-K on nutrient labels. These three elements serve major roles: nitrogen supports lush foliage and vigorous growth; phosphorus fuels root development and flowering; and potassium helps with overall plant health, water regulation, and resistance to diseases. You've probably heard these names tossed around, but what often gets overlooked is how finely balanced their levels must be through the different stages of growth.

In the vegetative phase, cannabis heavily demands nitrogen to build strong stems and abundant leaves. This is the stage when the plant is focusing on creating a robust framework, so ample nitrogen is key to vibrant greens and rapid expansion. However, once flowering begins, the emphasis shifts. The plant requires more phosphorus and potassium relative to nitrogen to encourage bud development and increased resin production. Feeding too much nitrogen during flowering can lead to leafy buds with less potency and a longer time to harvest.

While macronutrients take center stage, cannabis plants also require micronutrients—elements needed in much smaller quantities but no less important. These include calcium, magnesium, iron, zinc, boron, manganese, copper, molybdenum, and chlorine. Micronutrients often act as catalysts in enzymatic processes, facilitating nutrient uptake, energy transfer, and overall metabolic functions. Even a tiny deficiency can throw off a plant's health and result in symptoms like yellowing leaves, spotting, or poor bud formation.

Calcium and magnesium deserve special mention since they're often considered secondary macronutrients rather than pure micronutrients. Calcium strengthens cell walls, improving structural integrity and resistance to diseases. Meanwhile, magnesium is the central atom in chlorophyll molecules, making it essential for photosynthesis and energy production. Because of their importance, these nutrients are commonly added separately or included in balanced calcium-magnesium supplements, especially when using reverse osmosis water or hydroponic systems where these minerals may be absent.

One challenge many growers face is nutrient lockout. This occurs when the plant has nutrients available in the medium, but they can't absorb them due to improper pH levels or other environmental stresses. Lockout often mimics deficiency symptoms, causing confusion. That's where understanding not just the nutrients themselves, but how plants access them, becomes critical. Regularly monitoring pH and adjusting it to the recommended range for cannabis—typically between 6.0 and 7.0 in soil, and 5.5 to 6.5 in hydroponic setups—helps ensure your plants will take in what's offered.

Besides just quantity, the timing and ratio of macronutrients and micronutrients matter tremendously. Cannabis plants have shifting nutritional needs throughout their life cycle. For example, overfeeding nitrogen in flowering not only diminishes yield but increases the risk of pests and diseases, as overly lush foliage can trap moisture and provide hiding spots. Meanwhile, insufficient phosphorus during bloom can stunt bud growth and reduce cannabinoid production. Keeping balanced feeding schedules tailored to growth stages lays the groundwork for a fruitful harvest.

Another important aspect to consider is the nutrient source. Organic growers rely on natural amendments like compost, worm castings, bone meal, and kelp extract to supply both macro and micronutrients. These sources slowly release nutrients and improve soil biology, which can foster healthier, more resilient plants. Conversely, conventional growers often use synthetic nutrient formulations designed for quick uptake and precise control. Each method has merits and challenges, but in

either case, the fundamental need for proper macro- and micronutrient balance is unchanged.

Micronutrient deficiencies can be a bit sneaky. For instance, iron deficiency usually first shows in younger leaves with yellowing between veins, while zinc shortages cause distorted, stunted new growth. Boron deficiencies tend to affect expanding tissues and can cause brittle or malformed leaves. Recognizing these subtle signals early and responding with targeted supplementation can prevent severe problems that might otherwise reduce yield or damage plant health.

In understanding macronutrients and micronutrients, it's also helpful to recognize how they interact. Nutrients don't act in isolation; excess or deficiency of one can impact the availability of others. For example, too much potassium can interfere with magnesium uptake, leading to symptoms that look like magnesium deficiency even when magnesium is present. These complex interactions underscore why feeding cannabis is more than just dumping fertilizer; it requires attentiveness and nuance.

The physical environment also influences how plants process nutrients. Soil composition, moisture levels, temperature, and microbial life all affect nutrient availability and uptake efficiency. For example, in colder soils, root activity slows, which means nutrient absorption drops, so timely adjustments in feeding or environmental controls can help mitigate this. This dynamic relationship between plant needs and environment makes nutrient management a continuous learning process.

Finally, keep in mind that macronutrients and micronutrients don't just support growth; they influence the chemical profile of cannabis. Nutrient imbalances can cause a drop in the production of cannabinoids like THC and CBD, as well as terpene profiles that define aroma and flavor. So, maintaining a nutrient plan that meets your plants' demands sets the stage for both quantity and quality.

Ultimately, understanding macronutrients and micronutrients arms you with the knowledge to nurture your cannabis plants skillfully. Whether adjusting feeding schedules, diagnosing deficiency symptoms, or tweaking pH for better uptake, these fundamentals build confidence as a grower and increase the chance of harvests that make all the effort worthwhile. Paying close attention to these essential nutrients at every stage keeps your crops healthy, productive, and rich in the qualities you're seeking.

Feeding Schedules for Different Growth Stages

Proper nutrient management is the backbone of any successful cannabis grow. Understanding how to feed your plants at each growth stage can greatly impact overall health, vigor, and ultimately the quality and yield of your harvest. Unlike many crops, cannabis has distinct nutritional needs that shift dramatically as it moves from seedling to harvest. Getting familiar with these feeding changes will empower you to provide exactly what your plants need when they need it most.

Early on, in the seedling stage, cannabis plants are delicate and require a careful, gentle approach. At this point, the primary source of nutrition should come from a mild, balanced nutrient solution or, depending on your growing medium, nothing at all for the first week or so. Seedlings are sensitive to nutrient burn, and overfeeding during this time can stunt growth or damage young roots. A diluted feed with a low concentration of nitrogen, phosphorus, and potassium keeps the seedlings happy. Many growers prefer to start with just water and then gradually introduce nutrients after the first set of true leaves develop.

As your plants enter the vegetative stage, their appetite grows significantly. This is the phase when cannabis plants focus on developing strong roots, stems, and lush foliage. Nitrogen (N) becomes a key player here; it supports robust leaf growth and chlorophyll production, which in turn drives photosynthesis. A feeding schedule during the vegetative phase typically calls for higher nitrogen levels, balanced with adequate phosphorus (P) and potassium (K) to support root and overall plant health.

Feeding frequency in vegetative growth varies depending on your growing setup and medium. Soil growers might feed every 7 to 10 days with a nutrient solution or amend the soil with organic fertilizers, while hydroponic or coco coir systems often require more frequent, lighter feedings throughout the week. Keeping an eye on your plants and adjusting based on their responsiveness is essential. Nutrient lockout or deficiencies can quickly emerge if the feeding schedule is too aggressive or too lax.

Transitioning into the flowering stage, nutrient demands shift yet again. At this point, cannabis redirects energy from foliage expansion to bud development and resin production. The most critical adjustment is reducing nitrogen levels while boosting phosphorus and potassium. Phosphorus supports flower formation and root strength, while potassium aids in metabolic processes and resistance to disease. A well-calibrated flowering feed enhances bud size, density, and cannabinoid potency.

During flowering, many growers switch to a specialized "bloom" formula designed with the right balance of nutrients to stimulate bud growth and maintain healthy plants through the final stretch. Feeding intervals may become less frequent but often with a higher concentration per feeding. Overfeeding during flower can encourage unwanted foliage growth or, worse, cause nutrient burn that compromises bud quality. Watching for signs such as leaf yellowing or curling will help you gauge if your schedule needs tweaking.

Just before harvest, a nutrient flush is a common practice among growers aiming for smooth smoke and better flavor. This involves stopping all nutrient feedings and giving plants plain, pH-balanced water only. Flushing helps clear excess salts and residual nutrients from plant tissues, potentially improving the taste and harshness of the final product. The timing of this flush is critical; typically, two weeks before harvest is a good rule of thumb, but this can vary depending on your specific strain and feeding regimen.

Every growing environment and strain can respond differently to nutrient schedules, so it pays to tailor your feeding plan to match your conditions. Start with the recommended feeding chart provided by your nutrient manufacturer, but adjust based on observation. Keep track of how your plants respond to feedings, and don't be afraid to scale back or increase nutrient strength according to their needs. Consistency is important, but flexibility will get you that extra edge in quality.

Some growers also incorporate organic feeding strategies such as compost teas, worm castings, or seaweed extracts, which can supplement or sometimes replace synthetic nutrients. These organic amendments often provide micronutrients and beneficial microbes that improve soil health and nutrient uptake, especially during the vegetative stage. Whatever route you choose, understanding the fluctuating nutrient needs at each growth phase is the key to nurturing healthy plants right through to a successful harvest.

Remember, cannabis is a living organism that communicates through its growth patterns and leaf health. Yellowing leaves early in the vegetative stage usually point to nitrogen deficiency, while spotting during flowering might signal a phosphorus or potassium problem. Watching for these signs and adapting your feeding schedule accordingly will save you from costly mistakes. Keep your feeding regimen clear, simple, and based on the demands of each development stage.

The feeding schedule is more than just a timetable; it's a dynamic process that evolves with your plants. Whether you are working with soil, hydroponic, or coco coir mediums, balancing the frequency, concentration, and ratio of nutrients tailored to seedlings, vegetative, and flowering stages will lay a strong foundation for outstanding cannabis quality. With careful attention to feeding schedules, you're one step closer to producing robust plants loaded with potent, flavorful buds.

Organic Versus Synthetic Nutrients

When it comes to feeding your cannabis plants, one of the most common and important decisions you'll face is whether to use organic or synthetic nutrients. Both have their followers and unique advantages, but understanding the differences can make a significant impact on your crop's health, flavor, and overall quality.

Choosing the right nutrient type can also affect your growing style, budget, and the environmental footprint of your cultivation.

Organic nutrients come from natural sources—compost, plant matter, animal byproducts, and mineral deposits—providing a broad spectrum of macro and micronutrients in forms that soil microbes can break down and release gradually. This slow-release nature can support steady plant growth and build a living, healthy soil ecosystem over time. Synthetic nutrients, in contrast, are chemically manufactured and designed to deliver precise amounts of nutrients in soluble forms that plants can absorb immediately. They offer convenience and control, especially in soilless media or hydroponic setups where nutrient balance is critical and more easily managed.

The appeal of organic nutrients largely rests on their connection to natural gardening philosophies. Many growers report that organically fed cannabis often delivers superior flavor, aroma, and smoother smoke quality compared to plants nourished solely with synthetic fertilizers. That's because organic nutrients encourage a complex network of beneficial microbes and fungi in the root zone, which can enhance nutrient uptake and even produce secondary metabolites that add to the plant's profile. On top of that, organic growing aligns well with sustainable practices, reducing synthetic chemical runoff and promoting soil regeneration.

That said, organic nutrient use isn't without its quirks and challenges. For starters, because nutrients are delivered in complex, less bioavailable forms, it can take time for soil microbes to mineralize them into plant-friendly nutrients. This means occasional nutrient deficiencies or slower plant response times, especially early in the grow or if the microbial ecosystem isn't well-established. Properly managing organic feeds often requires more attention to soil health, batch preparation, and feeding schedules to avoid locked-out nutrients. Plus, beginners might need to experiment with different amendments or compost teas to find a winning formula.

On the other hand, synthetic nutrients provide growers with an unmatched precision in feeding. Commercially available formulas are crafted to deliver exact ratios of nitrogen, phosphorus, potassium, and trace elements, making it easier to tailor mixes to specific cannabis strains or growth stages. This level of control helps prevent common issues like nutrient lockout and deficiencies. Synthetic feeds are generally more concentrated and consistent, so many growers appreciate how straightforward they can be to dose, mix, and maintain during a grow cycle tailored to rapid vegetative growth or heavy flowering phases.

However, synthetic nutrients can sometimes be too aggressive, especially if over-applied, leading to nutrient burn, salt buildup, or disrupted microbial life in the root zone. Without the buffering effect of living soil, synthetic feeds may also create imbalances in soil chemistry that affect long-term health. In hydroponic systems, where organic amendments aren't practical, synthetic nutrients dominate and allow growers to push plants toward high yields, but the final product's flavor and aroma might not match those cultivated organically.

For a cannabis grower keen on maximizing personal control and speed, synthetic nutrients offer a straightforward path. Mixing and application schedules are well-documented, and many nutrient lines come with specific charts for cannabis that cover all growth stages. That said, synthetic feeding often necessitates careful monitoring of runoff pH, electrical conductivity (EC), and salt accumulation to maintain plant health, adding a layer of technical work that novices may find intimidating at first.

Organic nutrients, meanwhile, appeal to those who appreciate a more natural approach and want to nurture the soil ecosystem alongside their plants. Many growers using organic methods swear by the improved terpene profiles and overall complexity in their buds. It also encourages patience and observation, rewarding those willing to invest time in learning about compost teas, microbial inoculants, and soil amendments. Such commitment can deliver truly satisfying results in flavor and smoothness but may require more trial and error before dialing in a system that works consistently.

It's also worth mentioning that mixing these two nutrient types—known as a 'hybrid' feeding approach—is an option some cultivators explore. For example, using organic base soils with occasional synthetic boosts during peak growth or flowering stages can provide both stable soil biology and responsive nutrient availability. While this method can offer a balance of benefits, it demands careful management and observation to avoid nutrient imbalances or microbial disruption.

Environmental considerations often push growers toward organic nutrients, especially if the goal includes sustainable cultivation. Synthetic fertilizers are energy-intensive to produce and may contribute to pollution via runoff if not managed carefully. Organic amendments, while slower to act, generally support biodiversity in the soil and can reduce a grower's environmental impact over time. This can be particularly important for cultivators growing in residential areas wary of chemical use or those aiming for an eco-friendly, natural product.

The decision between organic versus synthetic nutrients can also come down to the specific grow setup—indoor soil grows tend to benefit from organic approaches due to the thriving microbiome that can be sustained in the medium. Outdoor grows with natural soil conditions likewise often flourish with organic feeds, feeding the land as you grow. Hydroponic and soilless mediums usually require synthetic nutrients for precise feeding, since these setups lack the natural microorganisms present in soils to break down organic material.

Cost is another angle to consider. While organic inputs like compost, worm castings, and bat guano may carry a premium price, they can often be reused or supplemented with homemade amendments, compost tea recipes, and other sustainable materials. Synthetic nutrients, meanwhile, vary in price but tend to be economical and widely available, offering a no-nonsense approach for growers who want reliable results without the extra effort of maintaining soil biology.

In the end, the choice between organic and synthetic nutrients should reflect your personal goals, growing environment, and willingness to engage with the process. Are you after the rich, complex flavors that organic soils often provide? Or do you want the quick, measurable nutrient uptake and operational simplicity of synthetic feeds? Neither approach is inherently better—it's about finding the right fit for your grow style and desired outcomes.

For beginners and intermediate growers, it might help to start with organic nutrients if working with soil, as this can build a forgiving environment for plants to thrive. Synthetic nutrients are excellent for those wanting a more technical and consistent feeding regimen, especially in hydroponics or controlled container grows. Whichever you choose, getting familiar with the nutrient profile, feeding schedules, and plant responses will give you the confidence to optimize your cannabis cultivation and unlock your crop's full potential.

Understanding the roles and characteristics of each nutrient type will prepare you for deeper knowledge later, like optimizing feeding schedules and addressing common nutrient issues. By carefully selecting and managing your fertilizers—organic, synthetic, or a blend—you'll be a step closer to growing cannabis worth bragging about, from first sprout through to harvest.

CHAPTER 17
WATERING PRACTICES FOR OPTIMAL GROWTH

Watering cannabis efficiently means striking a balance—too much, and roots suffocate; too little, and the plant's growth slows down. It's crucial to develop a consistent schedule that matches your plant's size, growth stage, and environmental conditions, while also paying attention to the soil's moisture levels to avoid guesswork. Quality water with the right pH supports nutrient uptake, so always consider what's in your water source before watering. Keeping an eye on your plants' responses—like leaf turgidity and color—helps you fine-tune your approach, ensuring that each watering session promotes robust, healthy growth without stress or waste. Remember, mastering watering is one of the simplest yet most impactful steps to boost your cannabis crop's potential.

Understanding Cannabis Water Needs

Getting watering right is one of the most crucial parts of growing healthy cannabis plants. While it might seem straightforward—just give plants water when the soil feels dry—the reality is a bit more nuanced. Cannabis plants have particular water requirements that change throughout their life cycle, influenced by factors such as temperature, humidity, the growing medium, and the plant's stage of growth. Understanding these water needs isn't just about keeping plants alive; it's about optimizing health, growth rate, and ultimately, yield quality.

Water makes up a significant portion of the cannabis plant's structure—often around 80 percent of the plant's fresh weight—highlighting how essential it is. Through water, plants transport nutrients from the soil to their cells, cool themselves through transpiration, and maintain a firm structure. Without adequate watering, these processes slow down or stop, leading to stress or even irreversible damage. On the other hand, giving too much water can drown roots, reduce oxygen uptake, and invite root diseases. Striking the right balance is the key.

The amount and frequency of watering depend partly on the plant's growth stage. During the seedling phase, cannabis plants need less water, as their roots are small and developing. Overwatering at this early stage often causes as many problems as underwatering. In contrast, during the vegetative phase, plants ramp up water intake thanks to rapid leaf and stem growth. By the flowering stage, plants consume even more water, supporting bud development and resin production. This means your watering schedule has to evolve with your plants; there's no one-size-fits-all solution.

Environmental conditions also greatly influence water needs. If you're growing indoors under lights, the temperature and humidity will dictate how fast water evaporates from soil and transpires through leaves. Hot, dry environments increase water demand, while cool or humid spaces do the opposite. Outdoor growers face even more variability—wind, sun intensity, temperature swings, and rainfall all affect how much supplemental watering the plants require. Keeping a close eye on these factors helps prevent common watering mistakes.

Watering practices must also match the growing medium you're using. Soil, coco coir, hydroponic setups, and soilless mixes all retain and deliver water differently. For instance, soil generally holds more moisture and releases it slower compared to coco or hydro systems, which drain quickly and dry out faster. That means plants in coco or hydro need more frequent but smaller watering sessions to stay hydrated without risking root rot. Knowing how your chosen medium behaves is the foundation for building an effective watering routine.

It's also essential to recognize the visual and physical signs cannabis plants give when they need water. Drooping leaves are the most obvious indicator, but it's important not to mistake overwatering for underwatering, as wilted leaves can appear in both cases. In underwatering, the leaves tend to feel dry and crispy, while in overwatering, they usually look swollen and limp. Checking soil moisture with your finger or a moisture meter avoids guesswork and helps fine-tune when to water.

Understanding cannabis water needs means blending observation with science. Plants communicate what they need, but growers have to listen carefully and respond accordingly. Cannabis doesn't thrive on a rigid schedule but rather on flexible care adapted to its current conditions and stage of development. Mastering this adaptive approach can significantly improve plant health, minimize stress, and boost potency and yield.

Another factor to consider is the quality of water being used. While the quantity and timing of watering are paramount, the water's chemical composition affects nutrient uptake and overall plant health. Cannabis plants prefer slightly acidic water, usually in the pH range of 6.0 to 7.0 when growing in soil, and slightly lower for hydroponic systems. Out-of-balance pH can lock out key nutrients, causing deficiencies even if the plants' roots are sitting in plenty of moisture. Regularly testing and adjusting water pH prevents these issues and creates an optimal growing environment.

Hard water, which contains high levels of dissolved minerals like calcium and magnesium, can also impact cannabis watering strategies. While these minerals are necessary nutrients, excessive amounts can throw off the nutrient balance or cause salt buildup in the root zone. Filtered or reverse osmosis water, paired with diligent nutrient monitoring, may be necessary in areas with hard tap water to maintain a healthy root environment.

Closely tied to water quality and quantity is the importance of avoiding water-related stress conditions, such as root rot or damping off, which can devastate young and mature plants alike. Root rot thrives in poorly drained systems where water saturates the growing medium for too long. To prevent this, allow adequate drying time between watering and ensure containers have proper drainage. Over time, a consistently wet root zone suffocates beneficial microorganisms and invites pathogens, so maintaining a balance is vital.

Some growers worry that watering frequency depends heavily on pot size or plant size. While these factors matter—larger pots hold more moisture and bigger plants use more water—the best guide remains the feel of the root zone. Using a finger test, a moisture meter, or simply lifting the pot to check weight helps gauge when water is needed without over-relying on strict schedules. This intuitive approach also lets growers adjust watering based on weather changes or unexpected stress factors.

One misconception often encountered is the idea that cannabis plants can survive on minimal water, encouraging some beginners to underwater as a form of stress training. While mild water stress can sometimes trigger beneficial secondary metabolite production in certain plants, it's a risky approach for cannabis. Chronic underwatering slows growth, reduces yield, and weakens plants, making them more vulnerable to pests and diseases. Instead, it's better to promote healthy, consistent water availability while considering other training methods to boost potency.

Lastly, cannabis water needs vary with different strains and genetics. Some indica-dominant varieties are naturally more drought-tolerant due to their origins in harsher environments, while many sativa-dominant strains thrive with more frequent watering in tropical-like conditions. Hybrid strains fall somewhere in between. Understanding the provenance and characteristics of your chosen strain helps develop a watering plan tailored to its natural preferences, thus improving the chances of success.

In sum, the principle behind understanding cannabis water needs is balancing supply and demand while adapting to changing conditions. Regularly assessing your plant and environment, staying tuned to feedback from the root zone, and ensuring quality water supply set the foundation for thriving cannabis growth. With practice, you'll develop a feel for when your plants need hydration and how best to deliver it to maximize growth, health, and final bud quality.

Avoiding Overwatering and Underwatering

Getting the watering right is one of the most crucial skills any cannabis grower can master. Both overwatering and underwatering can stunt your plants' growth, reduce yields, and introduce problems that might take weeks to fix. It's a delicate balance, but with practice and attention, you'll develop a keen sense for what your plants need.

Overwatering is arguably the more common mistake, especially for beginners. When you give your plants too much water, the oxygen supply to the roots gets cut off. Roots need air as much as they need moisture to thrive. With constantly saturated soil, roots can suffocate, leading to root rot and slow nutrient uptake. The symptoms typically show up as drooping leaves, yellowing, and a generally sluggish plant appearance. At first glance, drooping can look like a thirsty plant, but the reality is quite the opposite. It's important to learn how to tell these signs apart early on to avoid compounding problems.

On the flip side, underwatering stresses cannabis plants just as much. If the roots don't get enough water, the plant will wilt, leaves will curl inward, and growth rates will plummet. In severe cases, underwatered plants can become brittle and may die back completely. Unlike overwatering, the soil will feel dry to the touch, sometimes even pulling away from the edges of the pot. A common challenge is striking the right watering interval, especially with different container sizes or soil types. Outdoor grows, for instance, often need watering schedules adjusted by weather and soil retention.

One helpful method to avoid both extremes is to monitor the weight of your pots. When a container feels light, it's usually a good indicator that the soil has dried out enough for another watering. Heavier pots indicate enough moisture remains. This approach requires some trial and error at first, but once you get a feel for the weights, it becomes second nature. Pair this with checking the soil's surface about an inch down; if it still feels moist, hold off on watering.

Another trick is listening to your plants. Healthy cannabis will respond quickly to proper hydration. Leaves will perk up after watering within a few hours, and you'll notice more vibrant growth daily. Conversely, a plant suffering from overwatering may stay limp or develop yellow spots despite fresh watering. Keep a close eye on these subtle cues.

Soil composition plays a vital role in how often you should water. Well-aerated, fast-draining soils dry out quicker, so they might need more frequent watering. Heavier soils, particularly those with lots of clay or organic matter, retain moisture longer, increasing the risk of overwatering. Choosing the right soil mix tailored to cannabis cultivation can alleviate many watering headaches before they start. Good mixes provide both water retention and aeration—just the right balance for root health.

The size and material of your pots are also factors. Fabric pots tend to dry out faster than plastic or ceramic ones due to better airflow. This can encourage more efficient root growth but means you might water more often. Regardless of the container, ensure there's adequate drainage to prevent water from pooling at the bottom. Standing water can quickly lead to root suffocation and disease.

Environmental variables, like temperature and humidity, affect how cannabis plants consume water. Hotter conditions increase transpiration rates, so plants will drink more. In highly humid environments, plants lose less water through leaves, meaning the soil might stay moist longer. Checking these conditions regularly can help you predict watering needs more accurately rather than relying on fixed schedules.

When you water, don't just splash water on the surface. Deep, thorough soaking encourages roots to grow downward in search of moisture, strengthening the plant. Light, frequent watering fosters shallow roots that dry out quickly, leaving plants vulnerable to stress. Make sure water runs through the drainage holes, indicating the entire root zone has been hydrated adequately.

Several growers find it helpful to keep a watering log, noting dates, pot weight, and plant responses. Over time, patterns emerge that clarify the ideal amount and timing for watering your specific setup. This kind of record has long-term benefits because even subtle changes in temperature or light cycles can shift water requirements.

If you suspect overwatering but aren't sure, it's best to let the soil dry out a bit before the next watering. This pause gives roots time to recover and oxygen to penetrate. However, be cautious not to swing too far into underwatering territory while waiting. Use your pot weight and soil checks here to strike a safe middle ground.

Conversely, underwatering can sometimes be trickier to diagnose because wilting can mimic other issues. Aside from dryness, keep an eye out for leaf edges turning crisp or brown. These signs indicate your plant is seriously thirsty and needs immediate watering. Avoid playing a guessing game in this stage; act quickly, but ensure watering is thorough and not just a quick spray.

Ultimately, perfect watering is a dance between science and intuition. Cannabis plants, like people, communicate their needs when you learn to listen carefully. Watching your plants daily builds confidence and increases your chances of catching problems early. Even tiny adjustments to watering routines can lead to healthier, more vigorous growth and bigger yields.

Remember, no two grows are identical. Your soil mix, climate, container choice, and even the strain will influence watering needs. The goal isn't perfection but consistency paired with responsiveness. The more you observe and adapt your approach, the better your cannabis thrives—turning your grow area into a lush, productive garden.

Water Quality and pH Considerations

When it comes to watering cannabis plants, the quality of the water you use can make a huge difference in the health and productivity of your crop. Even if you're perfectly on top of watering schedules and nutrient feeding, neglecting water quality and pH can cause nutrient lockout, stress, and ultimately stunt your plants' growth. Before you even think about how much water to give or when to give it, understanding what's in your water and how it interacts with your plants is critical.

First off, the source of your water matters a lot. Tap water is the most common source for many home growers, but it comes with pros and cons depending on your location. Municipal water is treated with chlorine or chloramine to kill bacteria and other microbes, which is great for human safety but not always ideal for plants. Chlorine can evaporate if you let water sit for a day or two, but chloramine doesn't break down as easily. Both chemicals can disrupt the beneficial microbes living in your growing medium, which are key for breaking down nutrients and supporting root health.

For those using well water or collected rainwater, mineral content can vary significantly. Well water often contains dissolved salts and minerals like calcium, magnesium, and iron, which plants need in proper amounts. But too much of any of these can lead to buildup, causing nutrient antagonism where some nutrients become unavailable. Rainwater generally has low mineral content and is slightly acidic, which can be helpful in many grow setups—though it sometimes has contaminants depending on the environment. Testing your water source for hardness and mineral content can give you a solid baseline to tweak your watering routine.

Speaking of tweaking, pH plays an enormous role in nutrient availability. Cannabis roots absorb nutrients most efficiently within a relatively narrow pH range. If the water's pH drifts too far out of this zone, nutrients become locked out and can't be absorbed even if they're present in the soil or nutrient solution. For soil grows, the ideal pH is typically between 6.0 and 7.0. In hydroponic or coco coir setups, the window tightens to somewhere around 5.5 to 6.5. Going outside these ranges increases the risk of deficiencies or toxicities, which show up as yellowing leaves, curling tips, or slow growth.

Maintaining consistent pH is easier said than done, though. Water pH can fluctuate depending on its source, and it can shift again after mixing in nutrients or additives. It's essential to measure pH regularly using a reliable meter or test kits. Adjusting pH involves adding acids or bases—like phosphoric acid to lower pH or potassium hydroxide to raise it—so having these on hand helps you stay within target ranges. However, you don't want to wildly swing the pH; small gradual changes work best. Overcorrecting can stress the plants and cause more problems than the initial imbalance.

High-quality water means more than just the right pH and minimal chlorine—it also means controlling dissolved solids. Total Dissolved Solids (TDS) or Electrical Conductivity (EC) measurements provide insight into how much mineral content your water contains. Cannabis plants do need minerals, but too many dissolved solids can salt up your soil or medium and affect osmosis, which is how roots take up water and nutrients. Keeping TDS or EC in check prevents root burn and ensures your plants can access their feed without problems.

Filtering water is a common method growers use to improve quality. Carbon filters are effective at removing chlorine, chloramine, and many chemical contaminants. Reverse osmosis (RO) systems go a step further, stripping almost everything out of the water, leaving it very pure but also devoid of beneficial minerals. If you use RO water, you'll need to supplement minerals back in to avoid deficiencies. Some growers prefer mixing RO water with tap water to balance purity and mineral content, especially if their tap water is high in salts or contaminants.

Another aspect to consider is water temperature. While not a direct quality factor, water temperature influences oxygen levels: colder water holds more oxygen, which roots love, while warm water can hold less dissolved oxygen and potentially stress the roots. Avoid using water that's too cold or too hot; ideally, keep it around room temperature—between 65 and 75 degrees Fahrenheit. This helps maintain a healthy root environment and supports steady nutrient uptake.

Let's not forget the importance of microbial life in your root zone. Beneficial microbes often thrive or die off depending on water quality. Chlorinated tap water can wipe out helpful bacteria and fungi, which your plants rely on for nutrient cycling and protection against pathogens. Using water that's been left to off-gas or passing it through filters can help preserve microbial populations. Alternatively, supplementing with microbial inoculants after watering introduces helpful organisms that rebuild and support the root ecosystem.

For those growing organically, water quality is especially crucial. Since organic growers often rely on living soils packed with microbes, any disruption caused by poor water quality can cascade into inadequate nutrient breakdown and poor plant health. Inorganic nutrient formulations might sometimes mask water issues, but organic grows reveal them clearly. Regular testing and adjusting your water source to suit your soil's biology becomes a routine—and valuable—practice.

Seasonal changes also affect water quality. In some areas, your tap water might be softer in winter and harder in summer due to varying source water or treatment methods. Rainwater changes too: spring rain tends to be more acidic, potentially lowering pH, whereas summer rain can pick up more minerals and pollutants. Monitoring water over time helps you anticipate these shifts and adjust watering strategies accordingly.

For growers using hydroponics or soilless mixes, water quality takes on even greater significance. Since nutrients are delivered directly in solution, any irregularities in water composition or pH show immediate effects. Water with too many salts or improper pH can quickly stunt plants or cause nutrient lockout. In these systems, consistent measurement and precise adjustments become your best friends. While it might seem overwhelming at first, developing a habit of checking and balancing your water will pay off with stronger, more vigorous plants.

One mistake beginners often make is ignoring the water they use, assuming all water is good enough. This can lead to frustration when plants show signs of deficiency despite adequate feeding. Testing water and adjusting pH is a simple step that prevents a lot of headaches. Also, keep in mind that the water that comes out of your faucet is not necessarily the water your plants see—once it sits in the soil or medium, its chemistry can change through interactions with organic matter and microbes.

Establishing a watering routine that includes water quality checks means your cannabis plants stand a greater chance of thriving from seedling to harvest.

Start by testing your source water for pH and TDS. Adjust the pH before supplementing nutrients to avoid skewed readings. Use filtration methods if needed, and consider letting treated water rest for 24 hours to reduce chlorine or chloramine levels. Follow this with regular monitoring to catch any fluctuations before they impact your plants.

Watering combines science and art. Paying attention to the subtle nuances of your water's quality and pH unlocks the full potential of your growing efforts. The goal is simple: provide your plants with clean, balanced water that supports healthy roots, efficient nutrient uptake, and vigorous growth. Once you master water quality, you'll see noticeable improvements in plant vitality and yields, making this a foundational step toward achieving high-quality cannabis at home.

Chapter 18
Training Your Plants for Bigger Yields

Getting the most out of your cannabis plants means actively shaping their growth through training techniques that maximize light exposure and airflow, ultimately boosting bud production. By gently bending and securing branches or strategically removing certain growth tips, you encourage your plants to develop multiple main colas instead of a single dominant one, which translates to bigger, denser yields. These methods, whether low stress or high stress, invite you to interact more intentionally with your plants, turning a passive growing process into an artful combination of care and control. The right training approach depends on your strain, setup, and goals, but mastering these techniques can dramatically improve your harvest without needing more space or complex equipment.

Low Stress Training (LST) Techniques

Low Stress Training, often shortened to LST, is a popular and highly effective method for cannabis growers looking to boost their yield without putting their plants through harsh physical stress. Unlike high stress training techniques, which involve cutting or damaging branches, LST relies on gentle bending and tying down of stems to encourage the plant to grow in a more desirable shape. This method is especially favored by both beginners and seasoned cultivators because it reduces the risk of plant shock and recovery time, allowing your crop to stay healthy and productive throughout its growth cycle.

The core idea behind LST is pretty straightforward: by manipulating the plant's natural growing pattern, you create a more even canopy that allows light to reach more bud sites. Cannabis plants naturally grow tall and develop dominant central colas, which can lead to uneven light exposure. When you spread out the branches horizontally and keep the canopy flat, you maximize light penetration and airflow, which plays a critical role in producing larger, denser buds. Plus, evenly spaced branches give you easier access to all parts of the plant for watering, pruning, and inspecting for pests or damage.

One of the great things about LST is that it can be started early in the vegetative stage when the plant is still flexible. Young stems are easier to bend without snapping, and the plant responds quickly to the new shape by growing more side branches and colas. The typical process involves gently tying down branches using soft plant ties, garden wire, or stretchy rubber bands to stakes or the edge of your grow container. As the plant continues to grow, you keep adjusting the ties and repositioning branches to maintain an open, uniform canopy.

Unlike pruning or topping, LST doesn't remove any growth points, which means you're not sacrificing potential flowering sites. Instead, you're encouraging your plant to multiply bud sites by stimulating lateral growth. It's a subtle but powerful way to improve yields without sacrificing plant health or slowing down your grow. By regularly training the plant to grow wider, you also reduce the risk of mold and mildew, since better airflow moves through the canopy.

When you start LST, it's important to be gentle and patient. Cannabis stems are surprisingly resilient, but bending them too far or too quickly can cause tears and damage. A good rule of thumb is to bend the stem gradually over a few days and secure it in place with soft ties. Avoid using materials that might cut into the plant's surface, as this can invite pests or diseases. Instead, use things like garden twist ties or soft plant clips, which provide enough hold without harming the stems.

It's also helpful to work in small increments. Don't try to manipulate the whole plant in one go. Instead, start with a few branches close to the main stem and gradually expand the training as the plant grows. This incremental strategy lets your cannabis plant adapt naturally while maintaining steady growth. Checking your plant daily to adjust ties and ensure no part is under too much tension is an essential part of this process.

One challenge many growers face when practicing LST is balancing the effort between control and freedom of growth. While you want to encourage horizontal spread, you also have to watch for signs of stress or stem weakness. Watch closely for any spots where the stem is becoming too thin or discolored, as this might indicate too much pressure. These weak points often need a bit of extra support or slower training to prevent breakage. In some cases, growers add small plant stakes right next to these delicate branches for additional support.

Another advantage of low stress training is how well it works in limited spaces, especially for indoor growers. Growing cannabis indoors often means you're restricted by height and space, so vertically stretching plants can be problematic. LST allows you to control the plant's height by keeping growth more horizontal, which fits better under grow lights or inside compact tents. This makes it possible to get bigger yields even when vertical height is a limiting factor.

There are also variations of LST that growers use, depending on their setup and goals. For example, some growers combine LST with a technique called "main-lining," which creates a symmetrical, manifold structure with equal-size colas. While main-lining involves a bit more initial cutting, the principle of spreading the plant evenly remains the same. Others may use LST along with screen of green (ScrOG) methods, weaving branches through a net to maximize the canopy's exposure to light and maintain an orderly growth pattern.

While LST is an accessible and effective method, it still demands consistency and attention. It becomes part of your daily or weekly plant care routine to check ties, adjust branches, and keep an eye on overall plant health. However, the payoff is well worth it. By investing this extra care early on, your plants will reward you with larger buds, more even development, and a more efficient grow space.

One helpful tip to make LST easier is to incorporate flexible training tools from the start. Soft garden wire, plastic-coated plant ties, or even silicone strips work great because they offer enough hold but stretch slightly as your plant grows. Using stakes or anchoring points within the pot or grow container lets you create custom angles and shapes without stressing the stems too much. Many growers also find it useful to mark the training schedule in a grow journal, noting when adjustments were made and how the plants responded—this kind of documentation can improve your technique over multiple grow cycles.

It's important to note that while low stress training is less risky than other training techniques, it's not a hands-off approach. Waiting too long to start training or neglecting your plants during this phase can reduce its effectiveness. Early intervention, careful tie placement, and gradual bend angles are key factors in ensuring your plants stay happy and productive.

One misconception about LST is that it's only useful for increasing yield, but it also contributes to better plant health overall. By opening up the canopy, you improve airflow, reduce hotspot humidity, and allow light to reach lower branches. These factors together significantly lower the risk of mold, powdery mildew, and pest infestations, which can all compromise your crop. LST encourages a healthier environment inside your grow tent or garden, saving time and effort in the long run.

In conclusion, low stress training is an invaluable technique for any grower aiming to maximize yield without the risk of damaging plants. It requires patience, subtlety, and regular care but delivers impressive results in terms of increased bud sites, healthier plants, and more efficient use of your grow space. Whether you're growing your first plants at home or refining your cultivation skills, incorporating LST into your routine is a smart move that aligns perfectly with the goal of producing high-quality cannabis.

High Stress Training (HST) Methods

When it comes to boosting your cannabis plants' yields, High Stress Training (HST) stands out as one of the most effective and transformative approaches. Unlike

Low Stress Training (LST), which gently encourages plants to grow in desirable shapes, HST involves intentionally stressing the plant through physical damage. This might sound harsh, but controlled stress triggers the plant's natural defense mechanisms, often resulting in stronger, bushier growth and an overall increase in bud production.

The fundamental goal with HST is to manipulate the plant's growth hormones, especially auxins, to redistribute energy and resources into producing more main colas rather than just one dominant tip. In simpler terms, by cutting or bending parts of the plant, you're essentially telling it to "work harder" in multiple areas, which leads to a more even canopy and maximization of your grow space.

One of the most popular HST techniques is topping. This involves cutting off the main stem's tip just above a node where branches emerge. The plant then redirects its energy to the two branches immediately below the cut, effectively doubling the number of main colas. Experienced growers often use topping multiple times during the vegetative stage to create a wide, bushy plant prime for an abundant yield. Timing is important—cutting too early or late can slow growth or cause excessive shock.

Another common technique closely related to topping is fimming, which stands for "FIM cut" (a mispronunciation of "FIM"). Instead of a clean cut removing the entire tip, fimming partially removes about 75% of the new growth tip. This causes even more branches to sprout compared to topping, sometimes resulting in three or four main colas instead of two. Fimming can be a bit trickier to master because its results are less predictable, but once dialed in, it gives you a fuller plant with more bud sites.

Super cropping is a more advanced HST method focused on stressing the plant by physically bending the stems until the inner fibers break without cutting open the stem. This technique encourages increased nutrient flow and hormone production in the bruised sections, ultimately making the affected branches stronger and more durable. Super cropping is particularly useful for strengthening major branches that will support heavy bud sites during flowering, preventing breakage under the weight of dense colas. Plus, the additional hormone production stimulates more vigorous growth overall.

One thing that's vital to understand is that high stress training methods will temporarily slow your plant's growth as it recovers. This is why timing HST correctly during the vegetative phase is crucial. You want to give your plant enough time to bounce back before it transitions into flowering. During this recovery period, your plant's root system and leaves work overtime to repair damaged tissues and adjust hormone levels, so maintaining optimal environmental conditions—like proper lighting, humidity, and nutrients—is essential.

When applying any HST method, hygiene is key to preventing unintended infections. Make sure your cutting tools are sharp and clean, preferably sterilized with rubbing alcohol to reduce the risk of pathogens. Also, be gentle when bending stems to avoid snapping—if a stem does break, you can often tape it up with horticultural tape and help it heal, but prevention is better.

Unlike LST which can be done repeatedly throughout the plant's life cycle without causing much harm, HST techniques generally require a more strategic approach. Overdoing high stress training can lead to stunted growth or even plant death, especially for less resilient strains or plants already dealing with other stress factors like nutrient deficiencies or pest problems. Observing your plants closely after HST is crucial; look for signs of rapid recovery and new growth. If your plant struggles, adjust your care routine or give it more time to bounce back before attempting further training.

While many growers swear by topping and super cropping to maximize their indoor grow yields, outdoor cultivators also benefit from HST. In fact, some outdoor plants might handle stress better due to natural conditions and a longer growth cycle, allowing for multiple training sessions before flowering kicks in. But keep in mind that unpredictable weather and pests outdoors might complicate recovery, so always factor in your environmental conditions when planning HST interventions.

Beyond yield improvement, HST methods can also influence the overall structure of your cannabis plant to better suit your grow space and lighting setup. Topping and fimming produce a wider canopy, allowing light to penetrate more evenly across bud sites, reducing the common problem of shaded lower branches. Super cropping can help create sturdier branches that hold up heavy buds without sagging or breaking, which keeps more of your harvest viable and attractive.

It's a good idea to combine HST with other training methods for best results. For example, after topping or fimming, you can still apply Low Stress Training techniques to gently bend and spread branches horizontally, further optimizing light exposure and airflow. This integrated approach tailors the plant's architecture to maximize photosynthesis and reduce hotspots where mold or mildew could thrive during flowering.

At its core, High Stress Training is about working with the plant's natural growth responses and harnessing them for your benefit. It requires patience, attention, and sometimes a bit of trial and error. But once mastered, you'll notice your plants delivering fuller, denser buds and a more controllable, efficient grow. Whether you're growing in a modest closet setup or a dedicated grow room, introducing HST can be a game-changer for your harvests.

In summary, high stress training methods like topping, fimming, and super cropping offer powerful tools to manipulate cannabis growth for bigger yields. They push the plant to grow more colas, create stronger branches, and develop a more favorable structure for light penetration. These techniques do stress your plants, so timing, care, and recovery are paramount. Used wisely, HST can elevate your growing game, turning average crops into standout successes.

Topping, Fimming, and Super Cropping Explained

When you want to maximize the potential of your cannabis plants, mastering some key training techniques becomes essential. Among these, topping, fimming, and super cropping stand out as highly effective high-stress training methods. While they may sound intimidating at first, these techniques are quite approachable once you understand their purpose and how to apply them properly. Each one shapes your plants in a way that encourages bushier growth and, ultimately, bigger yields.

Topping is one of the easiest forms of high-stress training to grasp and is often the first step most growers try. Essentially, topping involves cutting off the very tip of the main stem just above a set of healthy nodes. This forces the plant to stop focusing its energy on a single dominant cola and instead redirect growth hormones to multiple new shoots. As a result, you get several main colas instead of one central stalk. This naturally leads to a bushier plant with more bud sites, which is what all cannabis growers want.

The ideal time to top is during the early vegetative stage, usually after your plants have developed at least four or five nodes. This timing allows the plant enough energy reserves to bounce back quickly and capitalize on the redirection of growth. Be sure to use clean, sharp scissors or pruning shears to make a clean cut and minimize stress and potential infections. While it may sound harsh, topping is surprisingly safe when done correctly, and your cannabis plants will reward you with wider canopies and better light penetration across multiple bud sites.

Fimming is somewhat similar to topping but involves removing only part of the new growth at the shoot tip instead of the entire apex. The name "fimming" comes from "Fuck, I missed," hinting that it originated as a happy accident when growers tried to top a plant but only removed part of the tip. Unlike topping, which generally leads to two main colas, fimming encourages the growth of three to four or more new tops. For growers seeking more colas without drastically upsetting the plant, fimming can be a helpful technique.

You'll also want to perform fimming during the vegetative stage, right when your plant is actively growing new shoots. Just like topping, it requires using sharp scissors to snip the top growth, but instead of a clean cut across the stem, you pinch or cut off about 70-80% of the tip. This partial removal sends mixed signals to the plant that it compensates by creating several new growth points. The real beauty of fimming is its ability to generate a denser canopy and better yields without as much recovery time as topping.

Both topping and fimming are excellent tools for shaping your cannabis plants, but they're just part of the high-stress training arsenal. Super cropping, on the other hand, focuses on selective stress applied to the plant's inner tissues rather than cutting. It involves crushing or bending the stems just enough to break down the fibrous inner cells without snapping the outer skin. This "soft" injury triggers a healing process that thickens the stem over time, making it stronger and more capable of supporting heavy colas.

Super cropping is usually done once your plants have grown a bit sturdier but before they start flowering, often in the mid to late vegetative period. Using your fingers, you gently pinch and bend a branch until it feels soft or slightly brittle but still intact. The goal is to create small injuries inside, prompting the plant to redirect resources to strengthen the damaged area. Over the next few days, the stem swells, becoming more robust, which helps the plant better support larger buds without bending or breaking during flowering.

Applying super cropping strategically can also enhance light distribution within your canopy by allowing you to reorder branches for better exposure. When combined with topping or fimming, it becomes even more powerful since you're encouraging not only more colas but stronger branches capable of supporting the weight. Unlike topping or fimming, which remove parts of the plant, super cropping maintains all the foliage, allowing for continued photosynthesis and nutrient absorption.

The key to success with these HST methods lies in timing, care, and knowing your plant's limits. Overdoing any technique can stress plants excessively or slow growth, which is counterproductive. For example, topping or fimming plants that are too young or unhealthy can stunt them severely. Likewise, being too aggressive with super cropping can cause branches to snap completely or invite infection. Patience and gentle handling are essential to let your cannabis plants heal and adjust after training.

One benefit of topping, fimming, and super cropping that often surprises new growers is how each method can contribute to a more efficient canopy. Instead of having one towering plant that blocks light from the lower branches, these techniques shape the plant into a multi-cola bush, optimizing light penetration. That's huge when growing indoors where every inch of height and light counts. Outdoors, training plants this way prevents wind damage by creating sturdier branches and a low, wind-resistant profile.

You'll want to keep a close eye on your plants after applying these techniques. A brief slowdown in growth is normal, but if your cannabis remains stunted or develops unusual discoloration, you may need to adjust your care regimen or rethink the intensity of your training. Regular pruning of dead or unnecessary leaves combined with proper nutrients and watering ensures your plants bounce back stronger.

Topping, fimming, and super cropping aren't magic buttons that guarantee massive yields on their own. But they're foundational tools that work hand in hand with good lighting, proper feeding, and a controlled environment to unlock your plants' full genetic potential. Integrating these techniques gives you more control over plant shape and structure, making your grow space easier to manage and more productive overall.

When deciding which method to use, think about your goals and growing conditions. Topping is great for beginners who want a straightforward way to promote branching. Fimming is excellent when you want multiple tops but prefer less downtime. Super cropping is ideal once you're comfortable handling plants and want to increase branch strength without sacrificing foliage. Many successful growers blend all three during a grow cycle to fine-tune canopy architecture and maximize bud sites.

In summary, these high-stress training methods challenge your plants just enough to change their natural growth patterns for the better without causing lasting harm. The result? Bigger, denser colas, a more even canopy, and ultimately a more rewarding harvest. It's a hands-on approach that builds confidence as a cultivator and a deeper connection with your plants. With practice and patience, topping, fimming, and super cropping become invaluable components of your cannabis cultivation skill set, giving you an edge in producing top-quality buds.

Chapter 19
Managing Plant Health and Stress

Keeping your cannabis plants healthy isn't just about dodging obvious problems—it's also about recognizing the subtle signs when things start to go sideways. Stress can come from many angles: nutrient imbalances, light intensity, pests, or even changes in environment. The key is to stay proactive by routinely checking your plants for early symptoms like wilted leaves, discoloration, or slowed growth, so you can react before damage sets in. Prevention plays a huge role here; maintaining a clean grow space, using natural pest deterrents, and ensuring your plants get consistent conditions help build their resilience. Think of your plants like athletes—train them well but avoid pushing them too hard, because stressed plants are more vulnerable to disease and lower yields. The goal is to create a stable, nurturing environment that encourages vigorous growth while minimizing stress triggers, setting the stage for a successful harvest every time.

Identifying Signs of Stress and Deficiency

Understanding how your cannabis plants express stress and nutrient deficiencies is crucial for a successful grow. Plants can't tell you what's wrong, but they give off clear signals through changes in color, shape, and overall vitality. Catching these signs early on makes all the difference. By recognizing symptoms as they appear, you can intervene before the problem worsens or affects the final quality of your buds. This section walks you through the most common signs to look out for and what they could mean for your plants' health.

One of the most obvious indicators of stress or nutrient deficiency is the change in leaf coloration. Leaves might start yellowing, display spots, or develop discolorations like purple or brown patches. Yellowing often points to a nitrogen deficiency, since nitrogen is essential for vigorous, leafy growth. In contrast, purple or reddish leaves might indicate a phosphorus shortage, especially in cooler temperatures. If you notice dark or rusty spots, your plants may be lacking potassium, which helps with overall plant resilience and water uptake. It's important to remember though, that these colors alone don't always tell the full story—they come alongside other factors you need to observe.

Leaf shape and texture also serve as key cues. Curling leaves can mean several things: nutrient burn from overfeeding, underwatering, or exposure to heat stress. Leaves that claw downward typically suggest nitrogen toxicity, whereas upward cupping indicates heat or light stress. Wilting—even when the soil feels moist—can signal root problems or oxygen deprivation. Dry, brittle leaves may result from nutrient deficiencies or environmental stressors like low humidity. When these symptoms show up together, they help pinpoint whether the issue is nutrient-related, environmental, or possibly pest-induced.

It's also essential to keep an eye on new growth versus older leaves. Deficiencies often start at one stage first. For instance, nitrogen deficiency generally appears in lower, older leaves because nitrogen is mobile inside the plant; the plant shifts what little it has to newer growth. On the other hand, elements like calcium and iron are immobile, so deficiencies first show up in the newest leaves at the top. Spotting these patterns helps you diagnose which nutrient might be missing more accurately.

Beyond leaves, stems and branches can exhibit stress signals. Weakened or thin stems suggest a lack of strong structural nutrients or insufficient light. If stems become darkened or discolored, it might point to disease or pest damage. On the flip side, overly thick or swollen stems can indicate overfeeding or irregular watering.

Monitoring the vigor of stems gives you a broader sense of your plant's health beyond just the leaf surface.

Environmental stress factors feed directly into how your plant looks and behaves. Heat stress, for example, forces leaves to curl and turn yellow or brown along the edges, while light stress—too intense or too close—can bleach leaf tips or leave them crispy. Cold stress often slows growth and may cause purpling or dark spots. Even humidity can influence leaf texture and droopiness. Since many stress signs overlap visually with nutrient deficiencies, understanding your grow conditions alongside symptoms is vital.

Remember, stress doesn't always come from just one source. Sometimes your plants are battling multiple stressors at once—like a minor root issue combined with slightly harsh light conditions. That's why documenting your grow environment daily, along with nutrient feeds and watering schedules, becomes an invaluable habit. The more data you accumulate, the easier it gets to link a symptom to its underlying cause.

Finally, keep an eye on your plant's overall growth rate and bud development. Stunted growth or smaller, less dense buds often reflect ongoing stress or sustained deficiencies. With cannabis being such a sensitive plant, even slight imbalances can trim your yields. Consistent drop-offs in vigor are a red flag signaling something's off, even if the leaves don't scream it outright.

By systematically observing your plants' leaves, stems, and general growth, you'll gain the intuitive knowledge needed to spot trouble early. This sensitivity to plant health will empower you to troubleshoot effectively, adapt your growing environment, and optimize nutrient regimens. You'll find that plants often stabilize quickly once you address their specific needs, translating into robust growth and top-shelf buds. Practicing this form of attentive care builds confidence and moves your cultivation skills to the next level.

Next, we'll explore strategies to prevent common diseases and pests, often the culprits behind stress symptoms. But before that, mastering the art of identifying subtle signals from your plants lays the groundwork for strong, healthy cannabis throughout every stage of growth.

Preventing Common Diseases and Pests

When it comes to managing the health and stress of your cannabis plants, preventing common diseases and pests is one of the most crucial steps. Even the most carefully tended crops can fall victim to these challenges, and the consequences often range from reduced yields to total crop failure. The best approach is a proactive one—combining vigilance, good cultural practices, and integrated pest management techniques to keep your grow environment hostile to harmful agents.

Disease prevention starts with maintaining a clean and controlled growing environment. Whether you're cultivating indoors or outdoors, the presence of mold, mildew, fungi, and bacterial infections can quickly derail your progress. These pathogens thrive in warm, humid, overcrowded conditions, so managing airflow and humidity levels is your front line of defense. Using fans and proper ventilation, alongside regular monitoring, helps prevent pockets of moisture buildup that allow diseases to take hold. Choosing well-draining soil or a soilless medium free from contaminants also cuts down on risks.

Another practical tip is to always sanitize your tools and growing area before and during the grow cycle. Trimming scissors, pots, trays, and gloves should be cleaned thoroughly with isopropyl alcohol or an appropriate disinfectant. This simple habit reduces the chances of transferring fungi or bacteria from one plant to another. Avoid introducing new plants into your grow space without a quarantine period, since pests and diseases can hitch a ride on live plants, instantly infecting your entire setup.

Besides pathogens, pests are among the biggest headaches for cannabis growers at every experience level. Spider mites, aphids, thrips, whiteflies, and fungus gnats are common offenders. Each species has its quirks, but they all share one thing: they sap your plants' vitality and open the door to secondary infections. Inspecting your plants regularly with a magnifying glass helps catch infestations early, before tiny bugs multiply out of control. Look under leaves, near stems, and around the root zone for any signs of webbing, discolored spots, or tiny moving dots.

Physical barriers are sometimes underrated in preventing pest intrusion. Fine mesh screens over windows, sealing gaps in indoor grow rooms, and using sticky traps effectively reduce the number of invasive insects reaching your plants. If you're growing outdoors, companion planting with pest-repelling herbs like basil, marigold, and mint creates a natural shield that discourages many common pests from settling in your garden.

Biological control methods add another layer of protection by introducing natural predators or beneficial microorganisms into your system. Ladybugs and predatory mites are excellent helpers that consume unwanted pests like aphids and spider mites. These allies often keep pest populations at bay without causing harm to your plants or requiring chemical intervention. Similarly, biological fungicides containing beneficial bacteria and fungi can outcompete or inhibit harmful pathogens, establishing a healthy microbial balance around your cannabis roots and foliage.

While chemical pesticides might come to mind as a quick fix, they're usually not the best solution in cannabis cultivation, particularly for home growers aiming for clean, potent buds. Many conventional pesticides can leave residues, affect terpene profiles, or even cause stress that reduces plant vigor. Instead, organic treatments—like neem oil, insecticidal soaps, and garlic or pepper-based sprays—are safer alternatives. Use these carefully and as a last resort, because overapplication can disrupt beneficial insect populations and harm your plants.

Good cultural practices tie it all together. Avoid overcrowding your plants to improve air circulation; dense foliage traps humidity and creates perfect conditions for mold and powdery mildew. Regularly remove dead leaves and debris from your grow area to eliminate breeding grounds for pests and disease. Balancing watering schedules to prevent waterlogged soil helps reduce root rot and other issues tied to excess moisture. Many growers find that meticulous cleanliness and routine inspection prevent problems before they escalate.

Environmental stress often opens the door to pests and disease, too. Plants weakened by nutrient deficiencies, improper pH, or erratic temperature swings are more susceptible because their immune responses aren't operating optimally. Maintaining stable, ideal conditions for your particular cannabis strain is essential not only for healthy growth but for resistance against invaders. This includes following proper fertilization schedules, ensuring consistent lighting, and monitoring your grow space's temperature and humidity closely.

Quarantine is an especially effective practice when introducing new clones or seeds. Keeping new material separate for at least a week gives you time to observe any pest activity or disease symptoms before exposing your entire crop. Many growers avoid moving plants directly from one grow area to another without this precaution, significantly reducing the risk of widespread infestations. During quarantine, treat any observed issues promptly to avoid contamination.

At its core, successful prevention requires you to know your enemy. Familiarize yourself with the signs of common cannabis pests like minute webbing from spider mites or the sticky honeydew left by aphids. Also, study symptoms of frequent diseases such as powdery mildew's characteristic white fungal coating or the gray fuzzy mold of botrytis. The sooner you recognize these early warning signs, the quicker you can act to stop spread and damage.

Technology can lend a hand, too. Many growers use apps and digital tools to track humidity, temperature, and light levels constantly, setting alarms for out-of-range readings that may promote disease or pest outbreak. Regular photographs and journals documenting plant appearance and growth progress make it easier to spot subtle changes over time. This level of attention can often mean catching problems before they make a significant impact.

Ultimately, preventing common diseases and pests is about maintaining a mindset of vigilance and control. Instead of waiting until symptoms appear, treat your grow environment like a carefully managed ecosystem, where every factor from cleanliness to plant spacing plays a role in keeping your cannabis healthy and stress-free. By incorporating prevention techniques early and consistently, you set yourself up to enjoy robust growth, bigger harvests, and buds that deliver the full quality and potency you've been working for.

Using Natural Remedies and Preventative Measures

Managing plant health is a crucial part of any cannabis grower's journey, and relying on natural remedies alongside preventative measures can be a game changer. Instead of jumping straight to chemical pesticides or synthetic treatments, using organic approaches not only protects your plants but keeps the environment and the final product safer. Think of it as building a strong defense system for your cannabis garden—one that discourages pests and diseases without introducing harmful substances.

One key principle is to focus on prevention before problems even arise. Healthy plants are naturally more resilient, so maintaining proper growing conditions like balanced watering, adequate light, and good airflow greatly reduces stress and vulnerability. When plants are thriving, they're less attractive to pests looking for weak hosts. This preventative mindset saves time and effort down the line, letting you enjoy a smoother growing experience.

Using companion planting is a perfect example of a natural preventative strategy. Certain herbs and flowers such as basil, marigold, and chamomile can repel common cannabis pests like aphids and spider mites. You can interplant these companions directly into your grow area or containers. This ecological approach not only discourages pests but also promotes biodiversity, encouraging beneficial insects like ladybugs and predatory wasps that naturally control harmful pests.

For pest management, neem oil is one of the most popular natural remedies. Extracted from the neem tree, it has insecticidal properties that target a variety of pests without damaging your plants or beneficial insects when used correctly. Neem oil also exhibits antifungal qualities, which help prevent issues like powdery mildew. It's best applied as a foliar spray during early morning or late afternoon to avoid leaf burn. Consistently applying neem oil, especially during the early stages of plant growth, acts as a protective shield to keep common invaders at bay.

Another effective natural treatment is insecticidal soap, which works by disrupting the cell membranes of small insects such as aphids and whiteflies. It's gentle on plants but tough on pests, making it a reliable go-to for organic gardening. Be sure to test any spray on a small section of the plant first just to check for sensitivity. Reapplication every few days might be necessary to fully remove the infestation, but used properly, insecticidal soaps usually don't harm your beneficial bug population.

Biological controls introduce living organisms that naturally target and consume pests. For example, releasing predatory mites can bring problematic spider mite populations under control, while lady beetles feast on aphids. These natural predators integrate into your grow environment, offering a sustainable way to balance pest populations without resorting to chemicals. They are especially suited for indoor and greenhouse grows where introducing natural predators is more manageable.

When it comes to fungal problems, natural remedies shine once again. Baking soda mixed with water creates a simple homemade fungicide that can help prevent and control powdery mildew. This mixture changes the pH on the leaf surface, making it inhospitable for fungal spores. However, it's important to apply it carefully and not overuse it, as too much baking soda can cause leaf damage. Consistency and moderation are key.

Garlic oil is another versatile natural antifungal and insect-repellent treatment. Its potent aroma keeps many pests at a distance, and the antifungal compounds assist in managing mold and mildew threats. Using garlic oil sprays regularly can help maintain a healthy microbial balance on your plant foliage and soil surface, further reducing disease risk.

One of the simplest yet most overlooked preventative steps involves good sanitation in your grow space. Removing dead leaves, trimming excess leaves to improve airflow, and regularly cleaning tools and surfaces cuts down potential breeding grounds for pests and pathogens. Keeping your grow area tidy plays a big role in maintaining plant health. Invest time in these regular maintenance routines to avoid unnecessary setbacks with your crop.

Soil health also ties directly into natural plant defenses. Using organic compost and well-balanced nutrients creates a thriving environment for beneficial microbes and earthworms. These tiny helpers break down organic matter, improve soil structure, and increase nutrient availability. Healthy soil leads to stronger roots and more robust plants, which in turn fend off diseases and pest attacks better. Consider adding mycorrhizal fungi supplements as well—they form symbiotic relationships with roots, enhancing water and nutrient uptake while protecting against harmful pathogens.

Another preventative tool is maintaining proper environmental conditions like temperature and humidity. Molds and mildews love warm, damp, stagnant air, so using fans to circulate air and managing humidity levels within the ideal range helps discourage fungal growth. Particularly during flowering, it's vital to monitor these factors closely. Simple measures like opening vents or adjusting your HVAC controls can prevent costly mold issues.

Natural remedies often work best when combined and rotated. Relying on just one method can allow pests or diseases to become resistant or return with a vengeance. Alternating sprays of neem oil, insecticidal soap, and baking soda-inspired fungicides can keep your prevention strategy dynamic and effective. Observing your plants daily and catching problems early gives you the upper hand.

It's also important to remember that the plant's own immune system plays a role in its defense. Stresses like overwatering, nutrient imbalances, or light shocks weaken plants, making them more susceptible to infections. Limb trimming to remove damaged or infected growth not only improves airflow but enables the plant to redirect energy to healthy parts. Natural plant stimulants such as seaweed extracts and compost teas promote vigor and enhance resilience without burdening the plant chemically.

For indoor growers, quarantining new plants before introducing them to your established garden is a simple but powerful preventative action. This practice helps stop the spread of unnoticed pests or diseases from newly acquired clones or seeds. Even in smaller grows, this extra step pays off by limiting infestations early.

In outdoor gardens, providing physical barriers like fine mesh insect netting protects vulnerable plants from larger insects like caterpillars and beetles without resorting to sprays. Encouraging pollinators and beneficial insects by planting diverse flowering species nearby further supports natural pest control. Creating a mini-ecosystem around your crop offers a natural balance that can prevent outbreaks.

Finally, documenting and keeping track of what natural remedies work best for your specific grow environment allows you to refine your approach each season. No two grows are exactly alike, and continuous observation and adjustment lead to more consistent success. Combining natural remedies with good cultural practices empowers you to manage plant health holistically, promoting stronger plants, higher yields, and cleaner harvests.

Ultimately, using natural remedies and preventative measures aligns with a more sustainable and responsible approach to cannabis cultivation. By nurturing your plants with care and thoughtful defense strategies, you can achieve healthier growth cycles while minimizing risks. This harmony between prevention and treatment is key to unlocking your crop's full potential.

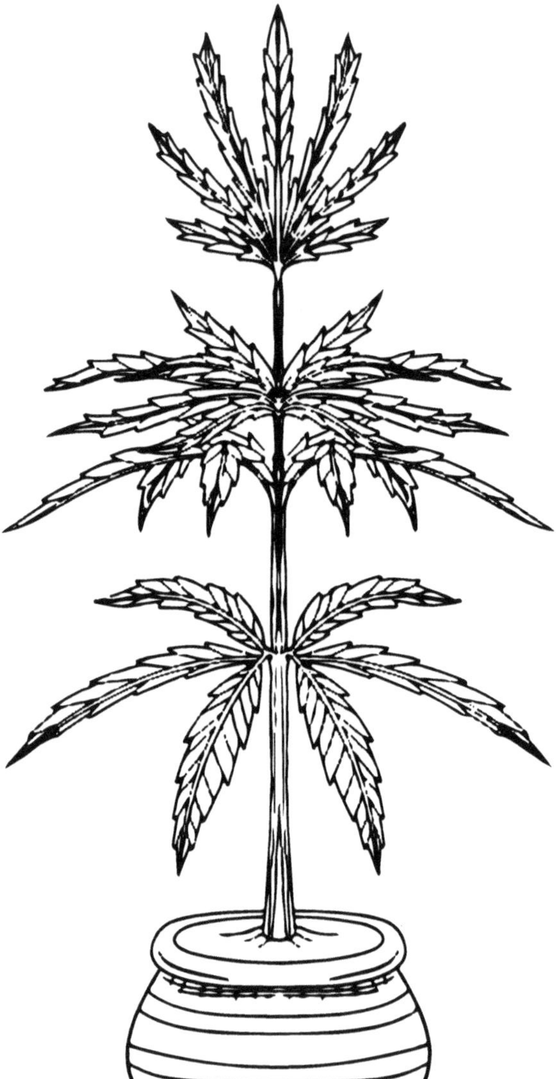

Chapter 20
Advanced Lighting Techniques

Lighting plays a crucial role in maximizing the quality and yield of your cannabis crop, and mastering advanced lighting techniques can take your grow to the next level. By understanding how different light spectrums influence plant growth and tailoring intensity to each growth phase, growers can stimulate stronger vegetative development and more robust flowering. Modern technologies like LEDs, HPS, and CMH each bring unique advantages, allowing you to customize your setup for energy efficiency, heat management, and spectrum control. Fine-tuning light schedules further enhances growth cycles, ensuring plants receive the optimal amount of light and darkness needed to thrive. Whether you're upgrading from basic setups or experimenting with lighting configurations, these strategies will empower you to push boundaries and cultivate healthier, more potent cannabis plants.

Understanding Light Spectrum and Intensity

When it comes to growing cannabis successfully, one of the most critical factors you'll want to understand is how light affects your plants. It's not just about having a light source overhead; the quality and quantity of light can drastically influence growth, health, and ultimately your harvest's potency and yield. To get the most out of your grow setup, especially if you're indoors, grasping the nuances of light spectrum and intensity is essential.

The term "light spectrum" refers to the range of different wavelengths of light emitted by your grow lights. Think of this spectrum as a rainbow laid out in tiny bands, each with its unique color and energy level. Cannabis plants respond differently depending on which parts of the spectrum they receive. While sunlight naturally provides a full spectrum, artificial lights vary widely in what wavelengths they cover. Understanding these differences allows you to mimic natural conditions or even tweak them to boost growth.

For instance, blue light, which falls in the shorter wavelength range, is key during the vegetative stage of your cannabis plants. It promotes strong, compact growth, encouraging the plant to develop sturdy stems and dense, broad leaves. In contrast, red light, landing at a longer wavelength in the spectrum, plays a vital role during the flowering stage, stimulating bud development and overall yield. By controlling the spectrum, you can guide your plants through their growth phases more effectively.

However, it's important not to think of light as just a simple on/off switch. The intensity of light matters just as much as the spectrum. Intensity refers to how much light energy your plants actually receive, often measured in micromoles per square meter per second ($\mu mol/m^2/s$). Too little light means slower growth, weak plants, and smaller buds. But too much intensity, especially without proper distance or adjustments, can cause light burn or stress your plants, potentially hampering growth or causing discoloration.

Light intensity decreases with distance—this is a fundamental principle many beginners overlook. If your light source is too far, your plants won't get enough energy to thrive. Conversely, if it's too close, there's a risk of scorching the leaves or overheating the canopy. Finding the sweet spot, based on the type of grow light and the growth stage, is a matter of monitoring and fine-tuning your setup. Remember, cannabis plants are living things that respond dynamically to their environment.

Besides the quality (spectrum) and quantity (intensity) of light, the duration of light exposure, or photoperiod, matters. Though this topic dives deeper into advanced light schedules, it's crucial to mention how spectrum and intensity influence the plant's internal receptors that detect daylight length. These receptors signal the plant when to switch from vegetative growth to flowering, affecting the final harvest timeline.

Modern grow technologies have made it easier than ever to dial in the perfect spectrum and intensity for your cannabis crop. LED lights, for example, offer incredible control because many models include adjustable spectrums and dimmable settings. This lets you customize your lighting environment throughout the plant's life cycle without switching out equipment or setups. While LEDs come with a higher upfront cost compared to traditional High-Pressure Sodium (HPS) or Ceramic Metal Halide (CMH) lights, their efficiency and flexibility often make them the top choice.

Another consideration when thinking about intensity is the footprint of your grow space. Intensity isn't just about power; it's about how evenly light spreads across your entire canopy. If some plants receive bright, direct light while others barely catch any, your harvest will be uneven. Balancing intensity and coverage means you might need multiple smaller light sources or reflectors to ensure all parts of your grow get sufficient exposure.

But remember, more light isn't always better. Cannabis plants have a limit to how much light they can process, called light saturation. Beyond this point, adding extra intensity won't increase photosynthesis and can potentially cause stress. Understanding this helps avoid wasting electricity and reduces the risk of damaging your crop. It's about quality energy delivery, not just brute force brightness.

Natural sunlight provides the best spectrum for cannabis because it covers the entire range the plant needs. However, for indoor growers, replicating this with artificial lighting requires careful selection and adjustment. Full-spectrum LEDs come closest by providing a balanced range of blues, reds, and everything in between. This balanced approach supports vigorous growth during all stages without forcing abrupt spectrum changes, which can sometimes shock plants.

Quality grow lights will provide a spectral graph, showing which wavelengths they emit strongly. This data is helpful when matching lights to your plants' needs. For instance, during early growth, focusing on lights with a higher output in the blue spectrum benefits vegetative development. When switching to flowering, a light source richer in red wavelengths optimizes bud formation. Committing to lights with a tunable spectrum gives you maximum control and often better results.

Intensity also changes naturally outdoors depending on the season and time of day. Indoor growers have the advantage of consistency but bear the responsibility for it too. Managing your light cycles and intensity carefully will mimic natural daylight rhythms your plants evolved to thrive in. This attention to detail creates healthier plants and superior harvests.

When setting up your indoor grow, a light meter or a quantum sensor can be invaluable tools. These devices measure actual light intensity hitting your plants and help you maintain optimal levels. They take guesswork out of how far to hang your lights or when to dim them. Regular monitoring ensures your plants are never too starved or overwhelmed by their light environment, allowing them to express their full genetic potential.

Understanding light spectrum and intensity also gives you an edge when troubleshooting growth issues. Yellowing leaves, stretched stems, or sparse buds can sometimes be traced back to lighting problems. Maybe your plants are reaching for light because it's too dim, or maybe they're showing leaf burn because lights are too close or too intense. Knowing the signs that point back to lighting helps you adjust quickly and avoid stress that can weaken your crop.

This foundational knowledge about light means you won't simply "turn on a light and hope for the best." Instead, you'll approach your grow room with purpose, selecting, positioning, and adjusting your lights based on scientific principles. Making these informed choices directly influences how robust your plants grow, how efficiently they use nutrients, and how thick and potent your buds become.

As you gain experience, keep in mind that light needs aren't static. Plants' requirements shift throughout their lifecycle, and the environment around them affects how they react to light. Factors like temperature, humidity, and genetics all play into how your plants absorb and use light energy. Pay attention to your plants' responses and be ready to tweak spectra or intensity accordingly.

Finally, this section sets the stage for more detailed guidance on specific lighting technologies and strategies found later in this chapter. Once you understand how light spectrum and intensity shape cannabis growth, you'll be better equipped to apply those insights using LEDs, HPS, or CMH lights. Each technology has quirks, but all of them follow the same fundamental principles outlined here, making the difference between average and exceptional crops.

In summary, mastering light spectrum and intensity is about more than just having a bright grow room. It's about delivering the right kind of energy to your plants at the right time, in just the right amount. When done well, your cannabis will flourish, producing potent flowers with rich aromas and strong yields. With this knowledge, you hold one of the keys to successful growing firmly in your hands.

Using LED, HPS, and CMH Lights Effectively

Lighting plays a huge role in the success of any cannabis grow, and among the top contenders are LED, HPS, and CMH lights. Each has its own unique advantages and quirks, so understanding how to use them effectively can make a noticeable difference in the health, yield, and potency of your plants. LED lights have surged in popularity thanks to their energy efficiency and customizable spectrum, while HPS (High Pressure Sodium) has been a long-time favorite for delivering intense, warm light ideal for flowering. CMH (Ceramic Metal Halide) lamps sit somewhere in between, offering a balanced spectrum that's closer to natural sunlight and often praised for promoting vigorous vegetative growth.

When choosing between these lighting options, the first consideration is your grow space and goals. LEDs tend to produce less heat, which is a big plus for smaller setups or anyone looking to minimize cooling costs. They also allow for spectrum tweaking, meaning you can optimize the light output for different growth stages. In contrast, HPS lights pump out high-intensity light that penetrates dense canopies well, making them a solid choice for larger flowering rooms where heat management is less of a challenge. CMH bulbs offer a middle ground in efficiency and spectrum completeness but usually require ballast compatibility and specific fixtures, so some upfront investment is necessary.

One key strategy for effective use is understanding the light spectrum each type emits. Cannabis plants rely heavily on certain wavelengths depending on their growth phase. For example, blue light (around 400-500 nanometers) is crucial during the vegetative stage for sturdy, bushy growth, while red and orange wavelengths (approx. 620-780 nm) spur flowering and bud development. LEDs excel because many units let you dial in these specific spectrums. Meanwhile, HPS naturally emits a strong red-yellow spectrum advantageous for flowering but weak in blue light, which is why some growers supplement HPS setups with metal halide bulbs during veg. CMH lights mimic more natural sunlight, offering a broader, well-balanced spectrum that supports plants throughout their lifecycle without additional supplements.

Proper positioning and distance of your lights can't be overlooked. Since LEDs typically run cooler, they can be placed closer to the canopy—often between 12 and 24 inches depending on wattage and model—without risking leaf burn. This proximity not only boosts light intensity but also encourages compact, resilient plant structure. HPS and CMH lamps emit a lot more heat, so they're usually suspended higher, around 18 to 36 inches above the tops of the plants, depending on fixture power and ventilation. Keeping lights too close to the plants can cause stress or bleaching, while sitting too far results in weak, leggy growth due to insufficient light. It's important to monitor your plants closely and adjust accordingly as they grow.

Managing heat is especially critical when working with HPS and CMH systems. These lights can raise the temperature significantly in your grow room, putting extra strain on your ventilation and cooling equipment. Implementing exhaust fans, air-cooled reflectors, or even air conditioning becomes essential in maintaining the ideal temperature range of about 68 to 78 degrees Fahrenheit for flowering plants. Not managing heat properly can stunt growth or exacerbate issues like nutrient deficiencies or pest outbreaks. LEDs, with their lower heat output, usually avoid these problems but still need adequate airflow to prevent humidity and heat pockets.

Energy efficiency is another aspect worth considering. While HPS lights have traditionally been favored for their low initial cost and proven performance, they consume more electricity and run hotter. That means higher energy bills and more money spent on cooling. LEDs tend to have a higher upfront price tag, but the energy savings and longer lifespan often balance that out over time. CMH bulbs fall somewhere in between: more efficient and longer-lasting than HPS, but less so than modern LEDs. If budget and sustainability are factors for you, these operational costs might tip the scales when deciding which lighting system to invest in.

Another effective tactic is to combine lighting technologies strategically. Some growers use a mixed setup, pairing LEDs with HPS or CMH to leverage the strengths of each. For example, LEDs can serve as supplemental veg lighting or for early flowering phases, while HPS lamps kick in heavy flower-stage energy. This blended approach maximizes spectrum coverage and intensity without committing entirely to one system's limitations. It also makes maintenance easier since you're not putting all your eggs in one basket. Just keep in mind that balancing light schedules and wattages becomes trickier with multiple fixtures, so careful monitoring is necessary.

Light schedules remain fundamental regardless of your lighting type. LEDs often come with timers or programmable features that make switching from veg (usually 18 hours on, 6 hours off) to flower cycles (12/12) seamless. HPS and CMH require external timers and sometimes manual adjustments. Proper timing directly influences hormones inside the plants, affecting flowering and overall growth rates. If the schedule isn't correct, stunted growth or hermaphroditism can occur, so keeping a consistent light regimen is key. The great news is, no matter which light type you deploy, modern technology has made staying on top of lighting schedules easier than ever.

One drawback of high-intensity lights like HPS and CMH is the potential for light burn or hotspotting. This happens when certain areas of your grow space receive excessive light, leading to heat damage or bleaching. Using reflectors and light diffusers can help spread light evenly across the canopy, ensuring all bud sites get quality illumination. LEDs often come with built-in lenses or adjustable angles that reduce hotspots, but it's still a good idea to observe how your plants react over time and reposition fixtures if needed. Uniform light distribution boosts photosynthesis efficiency and promotes even bud development, which translates to better yield and quality.

Replacing bulbs and maintaining your lights shouldn't be ignored either. HPS and CMH bulbs degrade over time, losing intensity and shifting spectrum balance, which can subtly undermine your grow. Typically, bulbs get replaced every 6 to 12 months, depending on use, to maintain peak output. LEDs, by contrast, last much longer—often five years or more—before their brightness declines noticeably. Keeping your fixtures clean and dust-free is also important since buildup can reduce light penetration. Regular equipment checkups ensure your plants are always getting the light they need.

Aside from tech specs, one crucial factor in using any lighting system effectively is closely observing your plants. Cannabis is remarkably responsive to light conditions, showing early warning signs when something's off. Leaves curling, yellowing, or bleaching can signal the light intensity is too high. Stretching or leaning toward the light source may indicate it's too low. Watching how your plants react as they move through each stage helps fine-tune your setup, ensuring that you're providing the optimal environment. Experience brings confidence here; every grow is a chance to learn and improve your lighting strategy.

Ultimately, successfully using LED, HPS, or CMH lights comes down to knowing their unique characteristics and tailoring your approach to match your grow room and plants' needs. Whether you're starting with a small closet grow under energy-efficient LEDs or managing a larger operation with HPS or CMH fixtures, mastering these lighting options gives you control over growth speed, health, and bud quality. With attention to detail and a bit of trial and error, you'll uncover what works best for your setup and enjoy the full potential these advanced lighting tools offer.

Adjusting Light Schedules for Growth Cycles

Lighting schedules are at the heart of successful cannabis cultivation. They directly influence how your plants develop from seedlings to fully mature buds, so understanding how to tweak these schedules across growth cycles is a game-changer. Whether you're growing indoors with complete control or supplementing outdoor light, adjusting light periods correctly can dramatically improve the health, size, and yield of your plants.

During cannabis growth, light schedules serve as signals that tell plants what phase they're in. These phases basically break down into vegetative and flowering stages. The timing and duration of light exposure essentially control the switch between these stages. That means, getting this right is one of the most critical steps for growers wanting to maximize quality and quantity. Just as importantly, improper light timing can stress plants, stunt growth, or even cause hermaphroditism, where plants develop both male and female reproductive organs.

Most indoor growers start with a "vegetative" light cycle—often 18 to 24 hours of light each day. This kind of extended light exposure mimics the long daylight hours of spring and summer, encouraging the cannabis plant to focus on strong stem and leaf development. In this phase, the plant is essentially bulking up and building the structure it'll flower on later. A longer light period ensures photosynthesis happens frequently, fueling rapid growth. However, some growers find that a full 24-hour light cycle can place unnecessary stress on plants that prefer a dark period to rest and respire, so 18 hours on and 6 hours off is often recommended.

After you've spent sufficient time in the vegetative phase with healthy growth, the next step is transitioning to the flowering stage. This is triggered by adjusting the light schedule to simulate the shorter days of late summer and fall. Commonly, growers reduce lighting to 12 hours of uninterrupted darkness and 12 hours of light daily. This shift signals the cannabis plant that it's time to start producing flowers (buds). Maintaining a consistent 12/12 schedule is essential because even brief interruptions in the dark period can confuse plants, causing them to revert to vegetative growth or develop hermaphrodite traits.

It can be tempting to immediately jump into flowering as soon as you see decent leaf growth, but patience here pays off. The vegetative phase sets the groundwork for robust bud development. Skipping this step or rushing can produce smaller yields and weaker plants. For most photoperiod cannabis strains, a vegetative period of 4 to 8 weeks is typical, but this depends on your strain choice and goals. Some sativas may need more time, while indicas often thrive with slightly shorter vegetative periods.

Autoflowering strains, on the other hand, operate a bit differently. They don't rely on light cycle changes to decide when to flower since this trait is genetic. With autoflowers, you generally don't need to alter light schedules drastically; many growers maintain 18 to 20 hours of light throughout the entire life cycle. That being said, understanding growth cycles is still essential because proper light intensity and duration affect overall plant vigor and potency, regardless of the schedule.

When adjusting light schedules, consistency matters more than anything else. Cannabis plants are incredibly sensitive to fluctuations in lighting—especially during flowering. Even short light leaks during the dark period can produce stress that leads to hermaphroditism or reduced yields. This is why using timers and light-proof tents or rooms is crucial. Make sure your dark period remains completely dark, with no artificial light sneaking in from outside sources such as streetlights or alarm clocks. Complete darkness ensures your plants receive an uninterrupted night cycle, which promotes healthy flowering and resin production.

Light intensity and spectrum also work hand-in-hand with schedule adjustments. For example, during the vegetative stage, your plants benefit from light that's higher in the blue spectrum, which fosters lush, leafy growth. When switching to flowering, shifting toward the red spectrum not only encourages bud formation but also complements the shortened light cycle. If your lights have adjustable spectrums or channels, coordinating light color shifts with your timing changes can push your plants to perform at their peak.

Not every grower follows the traditional 18/6 or 12/12 schedules exactly. Experienced cultivators sometimes experiment with slight tweaks, like 20/4 during veg or 11/13 for flowering, depending on strain-specific preferences or environmental conditions. These adjustments require close attention because small changes might mean the difference between a thriving crop and one riddled with stress symptoms. Starting with the tried-and-true schedules and gradually experimenting based on plant response is always a safer approach.

It's also worth mentioning the concept of "stretching" during the initial flowering phase. When plants first enter flowering after switching to 12/12, many experience rapid vertical growth for a week or two. This stretch can double or even triple plant height, which might be surprising if you didn't anticipate the jump. During this time, lighting height and intensity must be carefully managed to avoid light burn while still providing enough energy to fuel explosive growth. Anticipating and controlling this stretch can help you avoid overcrowding and optimize canopy size for better light penetration later on.

Adjustments to light schedules can influence not only growth speed but also resin and cannabinoid production. Cannabis plants produce more trichomes—the glands responsible for THC, CBD, and flavorful terpenes—when the light cycle induces proper flowering. Maintaining uninterrupted darkness in the flowering stage helps boost these compounds by mimicking natural seasonal changes. In contrast, inconsistent light cycles or light pollution can cause plants to reduce resin production to conserve energy.

When growing outdoors, light schedules are naturally governed by the sun's path, but indoor growers have the advantage of manipulating these conditions entirely. Additionally, some growers use supplemental lighting outdoors, particularly in northern climates with shorter daylight hours during parts of the season. Here, carefully timed artificial light can extend the vegetative phase or delay flowering, giving you more control over crop timing. Understanding how to tweak your setup accordingly can help you optimize yields even in less-than-ideal outdoor conditions.

Switching between growth cycles requires more than just flipping a switch. Keep in mind that when you alter the light schedule, plants take time to respond. You might not see immediate visible changes, but physiological shifts are happening under the surface. Patience is crucial as plants settle into their new rhythm. Hydration, feeding schedules, and environmental factors like temperature and humidity should be adjusted to complement the new growth phase and light schedule too.

Finally, regular observation and logging of plant responses after making light schedule changes are an essential part of mastering this technique. Tracking key signs like leaf health, stretch rate, and bud development will give you valuable data for future grows. Over time, you'll develop an intuition for how your specific strains react to different schedules, allowing for more precise adjustments that elevate your crop quality and efficiency.

In summary, adjusting light schedules effectively means more than switching timers; it's about understanding how light cues govern the plant's life cycle and using that knowledge to your advantage. With consistent schedules, careful timing, and close observation, you'll be able to direct your plants from seedling to harvest with confidence and success.

Chapter 21
Controlling Temperature and Humidity

Keeping the right temperature and humidity in your grow space is crucial for healthy cannabis plants and top-notch yields; too hot or too cold can stunt growth, while too much or too little moisture invites pests and mold problems. Each growth stage—whether it's the tender seedlings, the robust vegetative phase, or the delicate flowering period—has its own ideal environmental sweet spots to aim for, and maintaining those conditions consistently can mean the difference between a mediocre harvest and an exceptional one. It's worth investing in reliable tools like hygrometers and thermostats to monitor your setup, plus fans, heaters, or dehumidifiers to adjust conditions as needed to mimic nature's balance indoors or to complement outdoor climates. Mastering this element of your grow lets your plants thrive with less stress, making them more resilient and potent without the headaches of fluctuating or extreme environments.

Ideal Temperature Ranges for Each Growth Stage

Managing the temperature correctly throughout the cannabis growth cycle is vital for a successful harvest. Different stages of growth—seedling, vegetative, and flowering—demand distinct temperature settings to maximize plant health, development, and potency. Understanding these ideal temperature ranges helps growers maintain an optimal environment, preventing stress and boosting yields without wasting energy on unnecessary climate control.

Starting with seedlings, this phase is particularly sensitive. Young plants are fragile and rely heavily on consistent warmth to encourage steady root and leaf development. Seedlings perform best in temperatures ranging from 70°F to 78°F (21°C to 26°C). This range supports cellular activity without pushing the plant too hard, offering just the right balance to allow seeds to sprout strong roots and tender leaves. Temperatures outside this zone can slow germination or cause legginess, where seedlings stretch excessively trying to find light.

Humidity also plays a role here but we'll focus on temperature. When the environment is too cool, seedlings activate stress responses that limit growth or even cause failure to thrive. On the flip side, temperatures that climb much above 78°F risk drying the air and exposing tender tissue to heat shock, which weakens the plant's foundation before it matures.

Once your cannabis plants reach the vegetative stage, the temperature window shifts slightly upward with a bit more flexibility. The vegetative phase, characterized by rapid leaf and branch growth, thrives in a temperature range between 70°F and 85°F (21°C to 29°C). During this stage, plants benefit from higher temperatures during the light cycle, mimicking natural outdoor daylight warmth. You can afford to push toward the upper end of this range, especially when light intensity is high, because cannabis plants photosynthesize more actively in warmer climates during daylight.

However, temperatures near or above 85°F (29°C) require caution.

Excess heat can trigger stress hormones, slow nutrient uptake, or cause stomata to close as a defense mechanism, limiting photosynthesis. Nighttime temperatures should ideally remain about 5-10°F cooler than daytime temps to simulate natural fluctuations. This cooling helps plants recover and prepare for the next growth cycle. Maintaining these day-to-night temperature differences ensures vigorous vegetative growth and a healthy, bushy plant structure ready for flowering.

During flowering, temperature management becomes even more critical, not only for overall health but also for bud quality, potency, and aroma. Cannabis enters the flowering phase more sensitive to environmental stressors, and temperature swings can negatively impact resin production and cannabinoid profiles. The ideal daytime temperature for flowering ranges from 65°F to 80°F (18°C to 27°C), with 70°F to 78°F (21°C to 26°C) often considered the sweet spot.

Maintaining lower temperatures during flowering compared to the vegetative stage slows plant metabolism just enough to allow heavy bud formation while preserving delicate terpene compounds that define flavor and scent. Higher temperatures during flowering, especially above 80°F, can cause buds to become airy and less dense, diminishing final yield quality.

Besides daytime warmth, nighttime temperatures during flowering should drop around 5-10°F lower, usually settling in the mid-60s to low 70s Fahrenheit (18°C to 22°C). This drop not only mimics outdoor fall conditions when cannabis naturally flowers but also helps avoid mold and bud rot by limiting excessive humidity build-up inside the buds. Temperature control during this stage makes a tangible difference in harvesting sticky, potent flowers full of flavor and desirable effects.

It's worth noting that some growers find slight temperature variations within these ranges benefit strain-specific growth. For example, Indica-dominant strains can generally tolerate slightly cooler temperatures during flowering, while Sativas often prefer the upper range of temperatures due to their tropical origins. Hybrid strains usually adapt well within the recommended ranges but may lean closer towards one side depending on their genetics.

Even within ideal ranges, sudden temperature spikes or freezes can cause shock that sets the plant back days or weeks. That's why consistent monitoring and fine-tuning your grow environment with thermostats, fans, and cooling or heating units is essential. A gradual transition between day and night temps reinforces plant resilience and reduces stress symptoms such as leaf curling, discoloration, or slowed growth.

When growing indoors, artificial controls make it possible to maintain these temperature ranges more reliably than outdoors. Still, cultivators should prepare for seasonal changes or the heat generated by intense grow lights. Different lighting systems produce varying amounts of heat; for instance, high-pressure sodium (HPS) lights emit more heat than LEDs, impacting how you manage temperatures in your grow space. Understanding the heat output and adjusting ventilation accordingly helps you keep plants within their ideal temperature brackets.

Outdoor growers have the challenge of working with the natural climate, which requires selecting appropriate planting times or using shade cloths, fans, or heaters to buffer extreme weather. For example, planting early in spring or late summer may expose your crop to temperatures outside of optimal zones. Being aware of your local climate patterns and choosing strains suited for your region can also make managing temperature stress easier.

To summarize, the key to healthy cannabis plants is respecting their temperature needs at each growth stage. Seedlings like it warm but not hot, vegetative plants thrive in slightly warmer conditions that promote rapid growth, and flowering plants prefer slightly cooler but stable temperatures that encourage bud development without sacrificing quality. Adjusting temperature carefully across growth stages supports optimal photosynthesis, nutrient uptake, and metabolic processes that result in robust plants and quality yields.

Remember, temperature is never the only factor to consider, but it's one of the easiest to control and yields great rewards when managed correctly. By giving your plants this seemingly small but crucial advantage, you're setting them up for success every step of the way.

Managing Humidity Levels Indoors and Outdoors

Controlling humidity is a fundamental part of maintaining a healthy cannabis grow environment. Whether you're cultivating inside a carefully controlled grow room or out in the open air of an outdoor garden, understanding how to manage moisture in the air can make the difference between a thriving crop and one that struggles with disease or slow growth. Too much humidity creates perfect conditions for mold and mildew, while too little can stunt your plants and reduce resin production. Striking the right balance means you're giving your cannabis the best chance to flourish through all growth stages.

Indoor growers often have an easier time keeping humidity in check, thanks to the controlled environment of a grow tent or dedicated grow room. But even then, fluctuations happen. Activities like watering, plant transpiration, and ventilation changes constantly affect the moisture levels in the air. For outdoor growers, humidity management can feel more like a waiting game, influenced heavily by weather, seasons, and geography. Despite the natural fluctuations, there are still plenty of strategies available to improve your odds of maintaining optimal humidity.

Starting with the basics, cannabis plants have different humidity preferences during each growth phase. In the vegetative stage, they thrive at relative humidity (RH) levels between 40% and 70%. High humidity at this stage encourages healthy leaf and stem growth. As plants transition into the flowering phase, however, those humidity levels need to drop to around 40% to 50%. Lower moisture reduces the risk of bud rot—a dreaded fungal problem that can ruin an entire harvest.

For beginners, investing in a good hygrometer is essential. This straightforward device measures relative humidity, giving you immediate feedback on your grow space's conditions. Some models also combine temperature sensors, helping you monitor both critical environmental factors at once. Make a habit of checking your readings regularly; this will let you spot trends and nip problems in the bud before they get out of hand.

Inside, ventilation plays a crucial role in humidity control. Exhaust fans, intake vents, and oscillating fans work together to exchange humid air inside the grow room with fresh, drier air from outside, or at least redistribute air evenly within the space. Proper airflow also helps the plants transpire effectively by reducing moisture buildup on leaves. Without consistent air movement, moisture hangs in the air longer, inviting mold spores and fungus to settle in.

Dehumidifiers become an invaluable tool when you're chasing low RH during flowering. By pulling moisture directly from the air, these machines help maintain stable, precise humidity levels. This is especially important in climates or seasons where outdoor humidity remains stubbornly high. On the flip side, in arid environments or during winter months indoors, humidity can dip too low. That's where humidifiers come in, adding moisture back into the air and preventing your plants from drying out and becoming stressed.

Temperature and humidity share a close relationship. Warm air can hold more moisture, which is why you might notice humidity dropping as your grow room gets hotter under strong lights. Balancing these two is key for creating an ideal microclimate. For instance, running cool exhaust systems or air conditioners can reduce temperature and help manage humidity simultaneously, but if the air gets too cold, plants slow their metabolism and growth. Pay attention to how changes in temperature affect the humidity readings, and adjust your equipment accordingly.

For outdoor cannabis cultivators, the approach shifts slightly. You have less control over the environment, but you can still influence humidity through smart planning and plant placement. Choosing a location with good air circulation is critical. Avoid low-lying areas where moisture settles, like valleys or shaded spots trapped by surrounding foliage. Instead, opt for elevated spots or open areas with steady, gentle breezes to naturally reduce humidity around your plants.

Mulching your soil outdoors also affects humidity by regulating moisture evaporation from the ground. Organic mulches like straw or wood chips help retain soil moisture without saturating the air around your plants. This benefits root development while avoiding excessive ambient humidity that could promote fungal growth. Keep in mind, though, that when rain is frequent, you'll need to check underneath mulches for trapped moisture that might be too tempting for pests or mold.

Another outdoor tactic is selecting cannabis strains suited to your local climate's humidity patterns. Some strains naturally resist mold and mildew better and are more tolerant of fluctuating moisture levels. For example, varieties bred in humid, tropical zones often have thicker leaves and tighter bud structure, helping shed excess moisture. Researching strain genetics can save you from many headaches related to humidity stress down the road.

Monitoring outdoor humidity poses a different set of challenges. Portable hygrometers and weather stations can help you track conditions daily or even hourly. Integrate these readings into your cultivation routine to time watering and other interventions more precisely. Knowing when the humidity spikes—often at dawn or dusk outdoors—can guide you to take preventative steps, such as increasing airflow around plants or adjusting irrigation schedules.

Humidity's invisible presence makes it easy to overlook until it causes trouble like powdery mildew or bud rot. These issues aren't just cosmetic; they attack flower quality, potency, and ultimately, your yield. Catching early signs means inspecting your plants thoroughly and understanding how moisture accumulates on leaves, buds, and stems. If you spot a powdery white film or soft, dark spots forming, it demands immediate action.

Reducing humidity levels and removing affected parts can save your crop from further damage.

Indoor growers should develop a routine maintenance schedule for their environmental control systems. Clean fans, filter intakes, and dehumidifiers regularly to ensure peak performance. Dust and dirt buildup not only decreases airflow but also indirectly contributes to less effective humidity control. Automated controls linked to humidistats can automate this process, activating exhaust or humidification devices as needed to maintain your target RH without constant manual adjustment.

Even with perfect tools, environmental fluctuations happen. Outdoor conditions may change suddenly after a rainstorm, or an indoor sensor might read inaccurately if placed too close to a humidifier or watering station. Stay flexible and ready to adjust. Temporary increases in humidity can be offset by increased air circulation or shortening watering intervals. Similarly, when humidity dips, spritzing your plants with water in the morning can provide short-term relief, but it's not a replacement for proper equipment if low RH is a persistent problem.

Maintaining proper humidity balances also enhances nutrient uptake. When the air is too dry, plants close their stomata to conserve moisture, which restricts CO2 intake and slows photosynthesis. This stunted growth can manifest as nutrient deficiencies even if your feeding schedule is on point. On the other hand, high humidity can cause plants to become too relaxed, increasing the risk of nutrient lockout or other physiological stresses. Managing humidity is thus intertwined with every facet of plant health.

In the end, managing humidity is about creating a stable, predictable environment that mimics ideal natural conditions as closely as possible. For indoor growers, this means mastering your grow room's mechanics. For outdoor growers, it means working with the land, weather, and plant genetics to reduce risk. Both approaches require observation, patience, and a willingness to adapt your methods as conditions change. In doing so, you protect your crop from hidden threats and set yourself up for a bountiful harvest packed with quality, potency, and flavor.

Troubleshooting Environmental Fluctuations

Maintaining stable environmental conditions during your cannabis grow can be tricky, especially when external factors push temperature and humidity beyond the ideal ranges you've carefully set. Fluctuations happen—whether because of inconsistent HVAC systems, sudden weather changes, or even the natural heat produced by your grow lights—and these swings can stress your plants in ways that slow growth, reduce yields, or invite pests and diseases. Getting a handle on these ups and downs isn't just about fixing problems as they arise; it's about creating a resilient setup that minimizes disruptions and allows you to react quickly when things go off track.

One of the first steps in troubleshooting environmental issues is identifying the cause behind the fluctuations. Are your grow lights causing periodic temperature spikes? Could your ventilation system be inconsistent or undersized? Sometimes, external factors like hot afternoons or cold nights push the internal climate beyond your control if your setup isn't fully sealed or insulated. Knowing the source helps prioritize which tools or adjustments will have the most impact.

Temperature swings are among the most common challenges. Cannabis plants thrive within fairly narrow temperature windows—typically between 70-85°F (21-29°C) during the day and about 10 degrees cooler at night. When temperatures repeatedly go outside these ranges, especially with high heat during the light cycle, plants can experience stress that disrupts photosynthesis and slows overall development. On the flip side, temperatures that plunge too low at night can stunt growth and lead to issues like slowed metabolic processes or susceptibility to mold.

To address temperature inconsistencies, start by examining your lighting setup. High-intensity discharge (HID) lamps, for instance, generate a lot of heat and often cause spikes if placed too near the canopy without adequate ventilation. Switching to LED lights, which run cooler and are more energy-efficient, can drastically reduce heat buildup. Additionally, adding exhaust fans with temperature-triggered controllers ensures hot air is expelled promptly and replaced with cooler air. Using a thermostat-controlled heater or AC unit can also stabilize temperatures during cold nights or unexpectedly hot days.

Humidity fluctuations are just as critical to manage, if not more so. Cannabis plants prefer a relative humidity level of 40-70%, varying through their growth stages—higher during vegetative growth and lower during flowering to prevent mold and mildew. Problems arise when humidity swings rapidly, such as from overwatering or poor airflow, which can promote pests like spider mites or trigger powdery mildew outbreaks. Extreme dryness, on the other hand, leaves plants vulnerable to dehydration and slow growth.

If you notice wild swings in humidity, the first step is to check for moisture sources inside your grow area. Overwatering your pots causes excess moisture to evaporate, raising humidity unexpectedly. Ensuring proper drainage and watering only when necessary can cut down on this issue. Use humidifiers or dehumidifiers equipped with hygrometers and automatic controls to keep humidity steady. Good air circulation also helps prevent pockets of stagnant moist air where mold spores love to settle and germinate.

Another essential troubleshooting tip involves establishing a comprehensive monitoring system.

Relying on a single thermometer or hygrometer placed in one spot won't capture the varied microclimates that exist within your grow space. Instead, place multiple sensors at different heights and locations, especially near the canopy and close to the air intake or exhaust points. This way, you get an accurate picture of conditions across your grow area. Some growers incorporate smart devices connected to apps that send alerts when conditions drift too far from set thresholds, allowing fast response before damage breaks out.

Environmental fluctuations can also be a symptom of structural or equipment deficiencies. For example, poorly insulated grow tents or rooms are prone to temperature swings caused by external weather. Adding insulating materials or sealing gaps around doors and vents can make a huge difference in maintaining consistent conditions. If your fans or HVAC units are too small or underpowered, replacing them with more capable equipment may be necessary. Sometimes cycling your fans to run more frequently during peak heat hours is enough to smooth out the swings.

Be mindful of how plant transpiration affects your humidity levels too. When a dense canopy spreads out, the collective moisture the plants release can increase humidity, especially in smaller or less ventilated rooms. During flowering, when you want humidity lower to avoid mold, managing canopy density through pruning and training helps reduce the excess moisture output.

This also improves airflow, which is vital in preventing hot or humid pockets.

Occasionally, weird environmental fluctuations can indicate a failing or miscalibrated sensor. Always double-check readings from your devices against a reliable manual hygrometer or thermometer to rule out false alarms. Keeping your equipment clean and periodically recalibrated ensures you don't waste time chasing phantom problems.

When faced with a sudden spike or drop in temperature or humidity, react promptly. If your humidifier malfunctions and humidity climbs too high, instantly switching it off and cranking up your exhaust fan can prevent mold spores from taking hold. Similarly, if your room cools down unexpectedly due to a heater failure, turning on backup heat sources like small space heaters (with safety precautions) can prevent cold stress. Preparing backup systems and having emergency protocols in place for environmental control is essential for any serious grower.

Writing down daily readings and environmental changes in a grow journal may sound tedious, but capturing these fluctuations alongside plant responses helps you map out patterns over time. You'll start recognizing trends like humidity rising during watering days or temperature spikes coinciding with certain light schedules. This insight guides you to fine-tune your setup or timing to avoid recurring problems.

At the end of the day, troubleshooting environmental fluctuations is all about vigilance and adaptability. Cannabis thrives in balanced, predictable conditions, but perfect control isn't always possible. By knowing what drives temperature and humidity swings, implementing strong monitoring systems, fine-tuning your equipment, and staying attentive to your plants' signals, you create a more forgiving environment. That way, even when the climate throws a curveball, your crop stays healthy, vigorous, and primed for an abundant harvest.

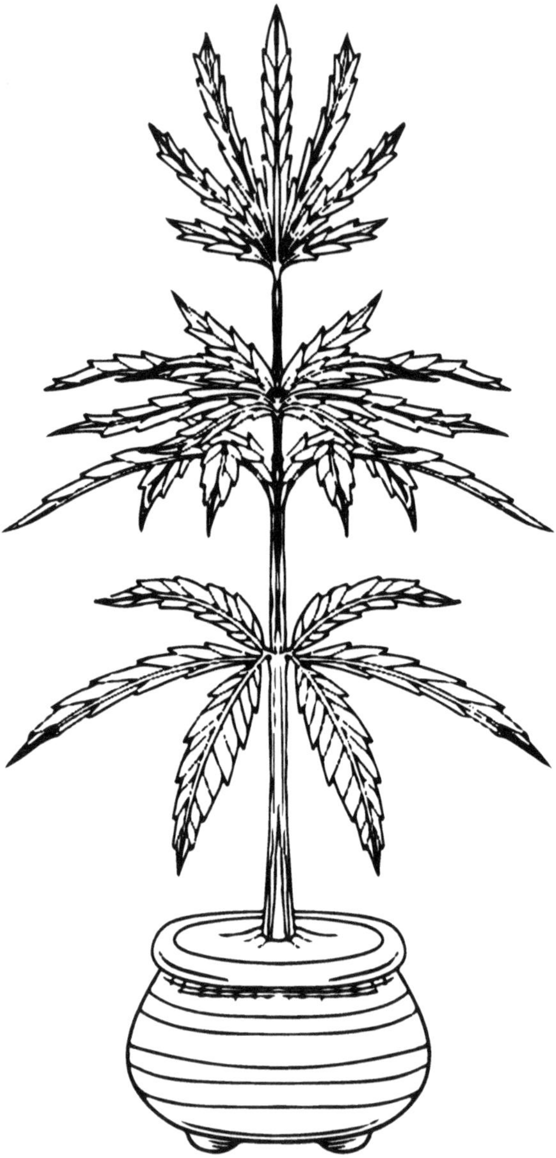

CHAPTER 22
HARVEST TIMING AND TECHNIQUES

Knowing exactly when and how to harvest your cannabis plants can make all the difference between a mediocre yield and a truly exceptional one, so it's crucial to pay close attention to the subtle signs your plants give as they near maturity. Observing changes in trichome color—from clear to milky to amber—and tracking pistil transformation help pinpoint the optimal harvest window, balancing potency, flavor, and effect. When it's time to cut, using clean, sharp tools and gentle handling preserves the delicate resin glands that hold your buds' valuable cannabinoids and terpenes, minimizing damage and oxidation. Proper harvesting techniques not only ensure maximum quality but also set the stage for effective drying and curing, which will be addressed further on, so mastering this step is key to elevating your craft and enjoying the fruits of your labor at their absolute best.

Evaluating Trichome Color and Pistil Changes

When it comes to determining the perfect time to harvest your cannabis, paying close attention to the trichomes and pistils is crucial. These tiny, resin-covered glands and delicate hair-like structures on your buds serve as natural indicators of maturity and potency. Learning to read their subtle transformations will help you know exactly when your plants have reached their peak cannabinoid and terpene profiles, maximizing both quality and effect.

Let's start with trichomes. These are microscopic crystal-like structures that coat the buds, sugar leaves, and even small stems. Their primary role is to produce and store cannabinoids like THC and CBD, along with terpenes responsible for the distinct aroma and flavor of your cannabis. As the plant matures, trichomes evolve in color and clarity, shifting from clear and translucent to a milky white, and finally to amber. Each stage tells a different story about cannabinoid development.

Early in flowering, trichomes appear almost glass-like. At this point, cannabinoid levels are still developing, and THC has not yet reached full potency. If you harvest during this phase, you'll get a milder, less intense high—often described as more energetic and cerebral. This may suit some growers, but generally, more patience leads to better results.

When trichomes turn milky or cloudy, the plant enters its prime harvest window. This phase indicates peak THC concentration, offering the strongest psychoactive effects. Cloudy trichomes mean the cannabinoids are fully developed but haven't yet begun to degrade. For many growers, this is the ideal time to harvest—especially those aiming for a euphoric, balanced high that doesn't feel overpowering.

As trichomes continue to age, they gradually darken to a rich amber hue. The amber coloration signals partial THC degradation into CBN, which has more sedative qualities. Harvesting with a higher percentage of amber trichomes usually results in a more relaxed, couch-lock effect. Some cultivators prefer a mix of mostly cloudy with 10-30% amber trichomes to balance potency with calming properties. Understanding your desired effects will guide exactly when you pull the trigger on your harvest.

Using a handheld magnifier or jeweler's loupe—ideally with at least 30x magnification—is essential for clear trichome inspection. Regular monitoring during the final weeks of flowering helps you track this gradual shift. Even checking your plants daily can make a significant difference in timing, preventing premature or late harvesting.

Alongside trichomes, pistils offer another vital visual cue. Pistils are the hair-like stigmas poking out from the calyxes of your cannabis flowers. Early in flowering, they are bright white and slender, signaling youthful growth. As your plants mature, these pistils darken and curl inward, turning shades of reddish-brown, orange, or amber. Their change mirrors the ripening process and complements trichome observations.

The transformation of pistils doesn't always follow a strict timeline or percentage rule, but a general benchmark is useful. When roughly 50-70% of the pistils have darkened and curled, your crop is usually approaching optimal harvest readiness. If most pistils remain white and straight, the plant needs more time to develop fully. Waiting too long after pistils darken can lead to overripe buds that lose potency and experience cannabinoid degradation.

It's important to note that pistil color isn't the most precise indicator by itself. Some strains naturally retain a higher percentage of white pistils even at maturity, while others darken quickly. Using pistil changes in combination with trichome color inspection provides a more reliable picture of readiness.

Experienced growers often keep a harvest journal, documenting trichome and pistil observations alongside environmental conditions and feeding schedules. This practice builds valuable reference points over multiple grows, helping you refine your timing and improve consistency in subsequent harvests. It's a simple habit that pays dividends for quality control.

Furthermore, environmental and genetic factors may influence trichome maturation and pistil coloration. Stressors like light intensity, temperature fluctuations, or nutrient imbalances can accelerate or delay these changes. Watching for signs of plant health during this critical phase ensures that delays or rushes in harvest aren't due to underlying problems. A healthy plant will produce vibrant, fully developed trichomes and pistils that are easier to judge.

When evaluating trichome and pistil progress, patience truly is a virtue. Rushing to harvest too early might yield buds with less potency and flavor. On the other hand, waiting too long could reduce THC levels, causing your crop to become more sedative than desired. Striking a balance based on your preferred effects and carefully monitoring these visual markers will give you the confidence to harvest at just the right moment.

Combining these observations with your own personal experience is key. Initially, it helps to take photos through your magnifier at different stages, then compare how the buds feel and affect you after drying and curing. Over time, you'll develop an intuitive sense of which trichome colors and pistil ratios match your ideal cannabis experience.

In summary, evaluating trichome color alongside pistil changes offers the most effective way to pinpoint harvest time. This approach centers on observing the natural indicators your plants provide. By honing these skills, you ensure that your homegrown cannabis hits the desired balance of potency, flavor, and effect—setting the stage for a successful harvest and exceptional final product.

Harvesting Methods to Preserve Quality

Once you've decided it's time to harvest, the way you handle your cannabis plants can make a world of difference in the final product's quality. Harvesting isn't just about cutting down your plants and calling it a day. It's a delicate, careful process that preserves potency, flavor, and the overall smoking experience. Knowing the best methods to minimize damage and degradation is key to ensuring that all the hard work you've put into growing your crop shines through in the final buds.

First and foremost, handling your plants gently is essential. Trichomes—those tiny, resinous glands packed with cannabinoids and terpenes—are fragile and can be easily knocked off or damaged by rough treatment. Bruising or squeezing your buds too hard when harvesting can cause resin loss, which lowers potency and diminishes that signature sticky feel many growers aim for. This is why tools and technique both matter so much. Choosing sharp, clean scissors or pruning shears to make precise cuts can really help reduce bruising and trichome loss.

Timing also plays into your harvesting methods. While the exact timing relates more to maturity indicators, once you spot the right window, harvesting more quickly yet carefully can reduce the risk of resin degradation from exposure to heat, light, or excessive handling. Some growers like to harvest during the early morning or late evening when temperatures and humidity levels are lower, protecting sensitive compounds from breaking down prematurely.

Another method to preserve quality is selective harvesting. Instead of cutting your entire plant at once, some growers prefer to harvest in stages. This method lets you focus on the buds that are perfectly mature while giving those needing more time a chance to finish developing. Sweating and curing benefits significantly from this approach, as it ensures that the buds you do harvest are primed for proper post-harvest care, while the rest of the plant continues maturing optimally. Selective harvesting calls for careful planning and bud inspection, but it can greatly improve your yield's overall quality.

Once you've cut your branches or whole plants, what happens immediately afterward influences quality just as much as the harvesting itself. Many cultivators recommend removing large fan leaves right away. This step helps improve airflow around the buds and reduces moisture retention, which can lead to mold if left unchecked. However, it's important to avoid too aggressive defoliation, especially around the delicate buds, since unnecessary handling can strip trichomes off the flowers.

During harvest, maintaining a clean environment is a subtle but powerful way to protect quality. Dust, dirt, and contaminants introduced at this stage can easily stick to sticky resin and cause issues during drying and curing. Wearing gloves and cleaning your tools between cuts reduces the chance of mold spores or bacteria hitching a ride on your buds. The goal is to carry your buds through every step of harvest and post-harvest with their integrity intact.

Some growers also employ a "wet trimming" method immediately after cutting, where the buds are trimmed while still fresh and wet. This approach can speed up drying by eliminating excess leaf material upfront, reducing the risk of bud rot. Wet trimming, however, generally requires careful quick handling to avoid damaging soft, sticky buds at this vulnerable stage. Others prefer "dry trimming," letting branches hang intact to dry before trimming, which can preserve trichomes better but needs extra patience and proper drying conditions to prevent mold.

Using the right tools and techniques for trimming ties directly into quality preservation. Scissors should be sharp and suited for precision cutting. Dull blades can crush or tear bud tissue, leading to resin spillage and faster degradation. Some growers even invest in specialized trimming scissors with tapered tips and ergonomic designs to help make clean cuts without fatigued hands. If trimming large quantities, it helps to take breaks to avoid rushed or sloppy cuts.

Temperature control during harvesting is another underappreciated factor. High ambient temperatures encourage terpenes to evaporate quickly, stripping your final product of some aroma and flavor nuances. It's best to harvest in cooler environments when possible or cool the room where you bring harvested branches for initial processing. This also slows down enzymatic reactions within the plant that break down cannabinoids and terpenes, helping preserve maximum potency.

A lesser-known but increasingly popular technique is the use of dark or dimly lit rooms during harvesting. Prolonged exposure to bright lights, especially direct sunlight or intense artificial light, can cause cannabinoids and terpenes to degrade faster. Working in subdued lighting minimizes this risk during the sensitive window between cutting and drying. This method is especially relevant for growers who harvest indoors where lighting might be intense otherwise.

Beyond handling and environment, careful planning of the drying setup immediately after harvest is crucial for preserving quality. Once your buds or branches are cut and prepped, they need to enter a controlled drying phase designed to remove moisture slowly without shocking the flowers. Rapid drying can lock in chlorophyll and other unwanted compounds, resulting in harsh taste and less pronounced aromas. Most growers aim for steady drying at temperatures between 60 and 70 degrees Fahrenheit with 50 to 60 percent relative humidity.

Good airflow without direct wind or fans blowing over buds helps prevent mold while avoiding scorching or drying the outer surfaces too fast. Hanging branches upside-down in a dedicated drying room or closet is the most common approach. It keeps the buds intact and prevents physical damage or crushing that could occur when laying trimmed buds flat. Maintaining a clean, dark, and well-ventilated drying space rounds out the set of methods that protect your cannabis' quality right after harvest.

Another noteworthy approach to maintaining quality during harvesting is the use of quick, low-stress movements. Moving rapidly but with control prevents unnecessary physical vibration or shaking that could dislodge precious trichomes. Experienced growers often develop a rhythm that balances speed with care, limiting the amount of time buds are exposed to air and handling while still avoiding sloppy cuts. It's a tactile skill refined over numerous harvest seasons, one that you'll grow into with practice.

Finally, how you transport your harvest to the drying area plays a crucial role. Avoid packing harvested branches too tightly in containers or buckets, since squeezing buds together can crush trichomes and encourage early degradation. Instead, opt for support methods like racks or breathable hanging nets that minimize contact and help maintain airflow during transit. The goal is to let your carefully harvested buds arrive at the drying stage in the best possible condition, free from mechanical stress or cross-contamination.

Ultimately, the way you harvest can elevate good buds into great buds. It's more than just a simple cut; it's a series of thoughtful steps designed to protect the delicate chemistry that makes cannabis special. Successful harvesting methods balance efficiency with gentleness—tools, timing, environment, and technique combine to preserve cannabinoids and terpenes, locking in the flavors and effects you cultivated throughout the grow cycle.

Preparing Buds for Drying and Curing

Once you've successfully harvested your cannabis plants, the next step is crucial: preparing the buds for drying and curing. This phase lays the groundwork for preserving potency, flavor, and aroma, so doing it right can elevate your final product from just okay to truly exceptional. While drying and curing get their own detailed focus later, this section zooms in specifically on what happens immediately after harvest to get your buds ready for those stages.

The key to preparing buds properly starts with gentle handling. Freshly cut cannabis branches can be delicate, and rough treatment risks damaging the fragile trichomes that contain most of the cannabinoids and terpenes. These tiny resin glands are what you want to preserve as much as possible, so always handle the buds by their stems and avoid crushing or squeezing the flowers themselves. Using clean, sharp scissors or pruning shears to trim the larger fan leaves away right after harvest can make the drying process easier and improve airflow around the buds, but avoid heavy trimming at this stage. Over-trimming too soon can slow drying and even rob the buds of some of their natural protection.

Another important consideration is deciding whether you'll dry your buds on whole branches or trim them into smaller sections before hanging. Both methods have their advantages depending on your setup and timeline. Hanging whole branches tends to slow down the drying process, which can be beneficial since slower drying often enhances flavor and smoothness. However, if space or equipment is limited, trimming your buds into smaller clusters or even individual buds can speed drying and reduce the risk of mold, especially in humid environments.

Once you've chosen your preferred method, pay close attention to your drying space's environment. Ideally, you want a dark room with temperatures between 60-70°F and humidity levels around 45-55%. This balance prevents the buds from drying too fast, which can cause the cannabinoids to degrade and the flavors to flatten. On the flip side, drying too slowly or keeping humidity too high raises the chance mold and mildew will develop. Before hanging, make sure your buds aren't wet or dripping with moisture. If rain or overwatering is a factor from outdoor grows, a brief air-dry period to wick away surface moisture can help.

Sanitation is another often overlooked, but essential part of preparation. Make sure all your scissors, knives, trays, and drying racks have been cleaned and sanitized beforehand. Introducing mold spores or bacteria at this stage can lead to trouble down the line. Also, if you're drying in the same space where you've been growing, it's a good idea to remove any plant debris or other organic waste to reduce contamination risks.

Trimming style during preparation also affects the drying and curing outcome. There are two common styles: wet trimming and dry trimming. Wet trimming involves removing most leaves immediately after harvest before the buds go into the drying room. This approach helps reduce the leaf material that slows airflow around buds and can speed up the drying process. Dry trimming, meanwhile, means hanging the branches intact and trimming after the buds have dried. This can preserve the shape of the buds better and prolong drying times, which many growers find improves taste and smoothness. Your choice should depend on your drying environment, patience, and preference for bud appearance.

Managing airflow in the drying room during preparation also matters. Proper air circulation helps wick moisture away evenly and prevents pockets of stagnant, humid air where mold might take hold. Using gentle fans set on low, placed strategically to move air without blowing directly on the buds, creates the best environment. Be careful not to overdo ventilation during preparation, or you risk drying buds too quickly, which can cause harshness and loss of essential oils.

It's worth mentioning how the timing between harvest and drying plays a role. Once buds are cut, the biological processes inside the flowers don't stop immediately. They continue to metabolize sugars and chlorophyll, affecting the eventual taste and smoothness of your cannabis. Preparing buds quickly and transferring them promptly to drying conditions limits unnecessary breakdown but doesn't rush things so much that you compromise trichome integrity.

In some cases, especially if you've grown outdoors, you might want to "wet cure" or do a quick rinse of the harvested buds before drying. This involves dunking the harvested branches or trimmed buds in water to wash away dirt, insects, or pesticides. If you do this, drying preparation takes on extra importance since the buds come out wetter than usual. Thoroughly drying the buds after rinsing and ensuring proper air exchange in your drying space prevents rot and mold from settling in.

Once trimming and hanging are done and your drying room conditions are dialed in, you're setting the stage for the 7 to 14-day drying window where the buds will slowly lose moisture while maintaining their potency and aromatic compounds. But before you get too far ahead, keep a close eye on the buds during the first few days of drying. This initial period is when the potential for mold growth or uneven drying is highest, so a quick inspection and gentle handling routine can catch early problems.

Finally, don't rush the preparation process. Taking the right time to trim carefully, set up the drying environment thoughtfully, and handle buds gently ensures the curing process will be smoother and more effective, preserving the quality you worked hard to cultivate. Each step from harvest to drying prepares your buds for that all-important final phase of curing where flavor and potency really blossom.

In summary, preparing your buds for drying and curing is a delicate blend of careful trimming, choosing the right hanging method, controlling your drying environment, and minimizing physical damage. This stage can seem tedious, but its impact on the final smoke quality is profound. Good preparation preserves your crop's hard-earned qualities and helps ensure you get the most from your grow, whether you're a patient beginner or a seasoned cultivator.

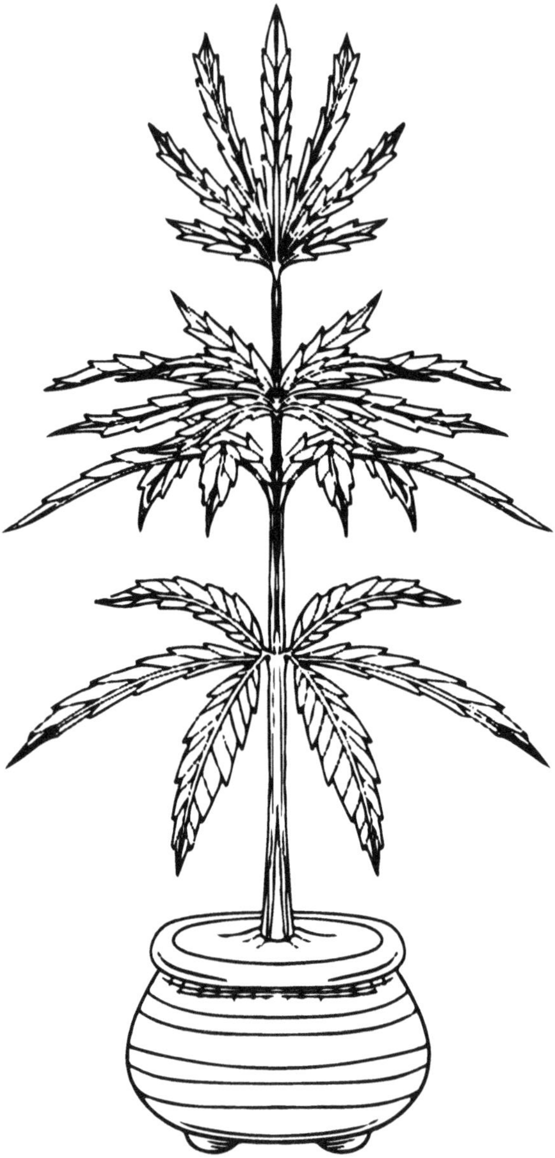

Chapter 23
Post-Harvest Quality Control

Once your cannabis harvest is secured, ensuring the highest quality doesn't end there — it's all about the details during post-harvest quality control. Keeping a sharp eye on drying room conditions like temperature and humidity can make or break your buds' aroma, flavor, and potency, so maintaining an optimal environment is crucial. This phase also includes careful monitoring for any signs of mold or overdrying, both of which can degrade your final product. Techniques such as gentle handling and consistent airflow play a big role in preserving delicate trichomes and enhancing the overall sensory experience of your cannabis. Troubleshooting common curing issues early helps avoid irreversible damage, setting the stage for a product that really stands out, whether you're sharing with friends or simply savoring the fruits of your labor.

Monitoring Drying Room Conditions

Once the harvest is complete, the drying phase becomes critical to preserving the quality of your cannabis buds. Properly managing the drying environment helps to lock in flavor, aroma, potency, and overall appearance. The drying room isn't just a place to hang your buds and wait—it's a carefully controlled space where temperature, humidity, and airflow work together to create optimum conditions. As cannabis enthusiasts and growers aiming for exceptional results, paying close attention to these factors can make all the difference between a mediocre stash and a premium product.

The first thing to understand is why controlling drying room conditions matters so much. When cannabis dries too quickly, the outer parts of the buds can become brittle and overly dry while the insides remain moist, leading to uneven drying and a harsh smoke. On the flip side, drying too slowly in a humid environment invites mold, mildew, and bud rot. Striking the right balance ensures that cannabinoids and terpenes remain intact while unwanted moisture dissipates properly.

Temperature is one of the most crucial variables to keep in check. Ideally, the drying room temperature should range between 60 and 70 degrees Fahrenheit. Temperatures above this range can cause the buds to dry too fast, which often diminishes terpene quality and can produce a harsh taste or smell. Lower temperatures, while seemingly safer, might prolong the drying and leave the cannabis susceptible to mold growth. Maintaining a consistent temperature is key because fluctuations can stress the buds and affect overall quality.

Humidity control goes hand-in-hand with temperature regulation. The ideal relative humidity (RH) for drying cannabis usually falls between 50% and 60%. This range allows moisture to leave the buds at a steady pace without drying out the surface too rapidly. Too low humidity can snap or crumble delicate trichomes, those tiny resin glands packed with cannabinoids and terpenes. Conversely, humidity levels higher than 60% create a breeding ground for mold, which can ruin an entire batch if not caught early.

Proper airflow is another essential piece of the puzzle. Good ventilation helps keep air moving smoothly around the drying buds, preventing pockets of stagnant air where moisture can cling. However, too much airflow directed straight at the buds can cause them to dry unevenly or become overly brittle. It's best to use fans strategically placed to gently circulate air throughout the room without blasting the cannabis directly. This way, moisture gets removed while protecting the buds' delicate structure.

Monitoring these conditions consistently is non-negotiable. Simply guessing or relying on occasional checks won't provide the precision needed to ensure excellent drying results. Many growers invest in digital hygrometers and thermometers that can log data over time, allowing them to spot trends and make timely adjustments. Some setups even include automated humidity controllers connected to dehumidifiers or humidifiers, creating an environment that self-corrects as needed.

Let's not forget about the physical layout of your drying room, which influences how well you can maintain these environmental factors. Keeping the drying space clean, dark, and separate from other grow areas prevents contamination and potential odor issues. Darkness is especially important because exposure to light can degrade THC and terpenes, lessening your final product's potency and smell. Hanging buds on clean racks or drying lines spaced adequately apart promotes good airflow and prevents overcrowding, which could trap moisture.

Another important tip is avoiding temperature or humidity extremes caused by the room's equipment. For instance, placing a dehumidifier or fan too close to buds might cause localized drying or stress to the trichomes. It's wise to experiment with fan speed and placement before the full drying process begins. Additionally, if you're drying a relatively small harvest, consider the room size and equipment capacity; overpowered systems can lead to rapid drying that's just as damaging as neglect.

As drying progresses over days or even up to two weeks, frequent checks are necessary. Simply relying on time alone won't assure you that the cannabis is drying right. Through touch and smell tests, you can gauge the drying stage—buds should feel dry on the outside but still a bit spongy to the squeeze and their aroma should become more pronounced as moisture leaves. If you notice a hay-like or grassy scent, it might mean drying has happened too quickly, signaling an adjustment for future cycles.

In cases where you catch signs of excess moisture or suspect slow drying, increasing airflow or lowering humidity slightly can help. Conversely, if buds feel too dry prematurely, raising humidity or slightly lowering temperature can slow the process. These subtle tweaks are what differentiate growers who consistently produce high-quality cannabis from those who settle for less. Remember, drying is not a static period; it requires active observation and adaptation to reach its full potential.

The payoff of carefully monitored drying room conditions extends beyond just smoke quality. Well-dried buds cure better and keep longer, preserving cannabinoid profiles and terpene blends. These compounds are what deliver the effects and nuanced flavors that cannabis lovers cherish. Proper drying also reduces the risk of contamination during curing and storage, making your cannabis safer to consume and more visually appealing.

Finally, embracing the responsibility of managing drying conditions cultivates a deeper connection with your harvest. It's rewarding to witness how attentive care during this phase elevates the work you've put into growing all along. Like any craft, mastery comes through understanding the science behind the process and listening to what your buds are telling you as they transform.

In summary, monitoring drying room conditions is an indispensable part of post-harvest quality control. Temperature, humidity, airflow, and room setup all play interactive roles in ensuring your cannabis dries evenly, safely, and optimally. With consistent vigilance and a willingness to adjust, you'll protect your buds' best characteristics and set the foundation for a top-shelf product that's well worth the effort.

Techniques to Enhance Flavor and Aroma

Once the cannabis plants have been carefully harvested and the drying process is underway, the next crucial step involves enhancing the flavor and aroma of your buds. This is where thoughtful post-harvest techniques truly shine. Flavor and aroma are carried primarily by terpenes—those volatile aromatic compounds that give each cannabis strain its unique scent and taste profile. But terpenes are delicate molecules, prone to degradation if conditions aren't optimized. This makes the post-harvest handling one of the most important phases for elevating your crop's sensory qualities.

One of the most effective ways to enhance flavor and aroma is to control the drying environment meticulously. The drying room should maintain a temperature between

60 and 70 degrees Fahrenheit and a relative humidity level around 55-65%. Too much heat will cause terpenes to evaporate quickly, dulling the aroma and flavor, while excessive humidity risks fungal growth. Keeping air circulation gentle but consistent prevents moisture pockets without stressing the buds. Many growers use small oscillating fans placed out of direct draft to maintain even airflow. It's a balancing act, but mastering it preserves those precious terpenes and cannabinoids.

Beyond environmental control, curing the buds properly after drying really unlocks their flavor potential. Curing involves placing the dried cannabis flower into airtight containers—often glass jars—and burping them regularly to release moisture and allow fresh air exchange. This slow process, which can last several weeks, lets enzymatic reactions continue that break down chlorophyll and other unwanted compounds responsible for harsh flavors or a 'green' taste. Gradual curing softens the smoke and intensifies terpene profiles, resulting in smooth, richly flavored buds.

Timing also plays a vital role during curing. Opening the jars for a few minutes once or twice a day in the first week balances moisture and prevents mold from forming. As the weeks progress, burping frequency can decrease, but the containers should remain sealed to lock in aromas. Many growers recommend curing for at least two to four weeks to see significant improvements, though some go even longer depending on strain and personal preference. Patience during this stage rewards you with a better tasting, more aromatic product.

Some cultivators experiment with natural additives to boost aroma during the curing phase. For example, adding a small piece of fruit peel—like orange or lemon zest—into curing jars for a day or two can infuse subtle citrus notes. However, these "infusions" must be done carefully to avoid introducing excess moisture or mold. Always monitor humidity closely and remove additives promptly. Another popular method is to use cedarwood or specialized cannabis curing packs that regulate humidity and impart mild woody or herbal scents. These tools manage moisture while enhancing olfactory complexity.

Temperature fluctuations during drying and curing can reduce taste quality, so keeping a stable climate throughout these stages is essential. Avoid exposing your cannabis to direct sunlight or heat sources as ultraviolet rays and excessive heat degrade terpenes and cannabinoids alike. Dark, controlled environments with consistent airflow maximize terpene retention. Some growers invest in specialized drying cabinets with adjustable climate settings, which takes the guesswork out of this critical phase.

Another technique to enhance flavor involves gentle handling of buds during trimming. Rough or rapid trimming can shake off trichomes and terpene glands, lowering the aromatic profile of your harvest. Taking your time to carefully trim by hand—not only preserves trichomes but also improves the visual appeal of the buds. Trimming just before curing (wet trimming) or after drying (dry trimming) depends on personal preference and strain type, but either way, precision matters to protect those fragile scent molecules.

Storing cannabis properly after curing also impacts the lasting quality of flavor and aroma. Using airtight containers kept in a cool, dark place helps maintain terpene integrity over time. Avoid plastic bags or containers, which can create static and degrade trichomes. Glass jars with tight seals remain the gold standard among enthusiasts. For long-term storage, temperature control becomes even more critical—think refrigerator or dedicated cool areas without moisture exposure to slow terpene breakdown.

Some growers swear by vacuum sealing and freezing their cured buds to "lock in" freshness. While freezing can preserve cannabinoids and terpenes for extended periods, it must be done carefully to prevent trichome damage from ice crystals forming. Using vacuum-sealed bags with minimal air and freezing in short bursts rather than prolonged periods is a safer approach. When you're ready to consume, thaw the cannabis slowly to avoid condensation, which could foster mold.

It's worth mentioning the importance of strain selection in your journey to maximize flavor and aroma. Some strains naturally produce richer terpene profiles, which respond best to ideal curing and drying conditions.

Indicas might bring earthy, spicy notes, while sativas often express citrus, floral, or pine aromas. Hybrids blend these characteristics and vary widely. Understanding your strain's terpene makeup helps you tailor post-harvest techniques for the best sensory results.

Innovative growers also explore terpene preservation through supplemental approaches like terpene-enhancing packaging or storage with terpene boosters. These products contain botanical terpenes designed to amplify specific scent profiles once stored with cannabis. While still niche, this technique highlights how seriously many growers take the art of flavor cultivation post-harvest. Combining natural drying and curing with such advancements can elevate even average crops into sensory experiences.

Lastly, maintaining strict cleanliness throughout the post-harvest process is essential. Contaminants and unwanted microorganisms can alter your harvest's smell and taste in undesired ways. Always sanitize tools, containers, and drying environments to reduce risk of mold, bacterial growth, or off-flavors. The goal is a clean, pure cannabis aroma unmarred by harsh chemical or musty odors. A hygienic workspace goes hand-in-hand with flavor optimization.

In summary, your cannabis crop's final flavor and aroma depend largely on a well-controlled post-harvest routine. Paying close attention to drying environment, patient and careful curing, gentle trimming, and proper storage are the keys to preserving and enhancing those precious terpene profiles. Fine-tuning these techniques helps transform your homegrown buds from good to exceptional, delivering rich sensory experiences that truly celebrate the essence of your labor. With practice and dedication, you'll find your prized harvests bursting with the full bouquet of aromas and tastes that every cannabis connoisseur seeks.

Troubleshooting Common Curing Problems

Once the harvest is in and your buds have dried, curing becomes the final but crucial step to unlocking their full potential. However, curing can sometimes be a tricky process, especially if environmental conditions aren't just right or if some details get overlooked. Even a small misstep can lead to undesirable flavors, harsh smoke, or worse, mold and mildew. Understanding how to spot and fix these issues early on is essential to preserving the quality and potency of your cannabis. This section digs into the most common curing problems you may encounter and offers practical advice to troubleshoot them effectively.

One of the most frequent issues growers face during curing is mold growth. Mold tends to develop when humidity is too high or when the buds aren't dried thoroughly before being placed in jars or containers. It often shows up as white, fuzzy patches or can sometimes appear gray or green. Catching mold early is critical; once it spreads deep inside the buds, it's nearly impossible to save your harvest without discarding the affected flowers. The best defense is maintaining perfect moisture levels—typically, humidity inside curing containers should stay between 58% and 62%. Using humidity packs designed for cannabis can help stabilize conditions and prevent mold outbreaks.

Another challenge relates to over-drying. While drying is a necessary phase before curing, if buds become brittle and crumbly too quickly, their terpene profiles may suffer, resulting in dull aroma and flavor. Overly dry cannabis tends to give a harsher smoke, robbing you of that smooth, rich experience high-quality buds are known for. If you notice your flowers cracking or turning powdery during the initial dry, it's a sign they were dried too aggressively or exposed to excessive airflow and heat. In these cases, it's helpful to slightly increase humidity during cure by using moisture control packs or temporarily "burping" your jars longer to rehydrate them gradually.

One subtle but frustrating problem is the uneven cure—where some buds inside the same jar cure perfectly, while others end up too moist or dry. This usually happens if your jars are packed too tightly without proper airflow or if the batch was mixed from buds dried at different rates. It's essential to be consistent with drying before placing buds in curing containers, and to avoid compressing cannabis too firmly inside jars. During cure, opening the containers daily (a process called burping) helps release excess moisture and refreshes the air, promoting uniform curing. If you spot that the moisture feels imbalanced, removing dense buds for a bit to dry separately can sometimes save the rest of the harvest.

Sometimes, growers might encounter an odd grassy or hay-like smell even after weeks of curing. This often results from insufficient or improper drying prior to curing, signaling that chlorophyll and other unwanted plant materials haven't broken down fully. While chlorophyll doesn't cause harm, it creates a harsher taste and can reduce overall smoothness. To avoid this, make sure your drying conditions are mild and controlled—too hot or too cold can interfere with proper breakdown of chlorophyll. If you catch this issue midway through curing, increasing the burping frequency and gently fluffing buds inside the jars can help gases escape and reduce that grassy aroma over time.

Temperature swings during curing can also throw a wrench in the process. Temperature influences how slowly or quickly cannabis cures—the ideal range typically falls between 60°F and 70°F. When temperatures climb much higher, the evaporation speeds up and delicate terpenes evaporate too quickly, diminishing flavor and aroma. Conversely, lower temperatures slow curing dramatically and risk mold formation if humidity isn't closely monitored. Fluctuating conditions stress the buds and make maintaining optimal humidity tougher, so stabilizing environment in your curing space pays off in much better end results.

Bud structure and density sometimes complicate curing as well. Dense, heavy buds trap moisture longer and dry at a slower rate, meaning they are more prone to developing mold if moisture isn't released regularly. Conversely, airy or less dense buds might dry too quickly and lose key volatile compounds prematurely. Adjusting curing practices according to your strain's characteristics is key here. Dense buds may require more frequent burping and careful monitoring, while lighter buds can benefit from slightly less airflow to avoid overdrying. Observing how your specific strain behaves and adjusting the curing schedule accordingly will improve consistency.

One of the most overlooked aspects of curing troubleshooting is the choice of curing containers. Glass jars remain the gold standard because they are non-porous and airtight, helping maintain steady humidity. Plastic containers or bags, on the other hand, can cause static, degrade terpenes, or allow too much air exchange, leading to faster drying or uneven curing. If you face issues with mold or pests during cure, switching to high-quality glass jars can make a notable difference. Also, avoid resealing jars immediately after opening during burping; letting air circulate for several minutes each day allows trapped moisture and gases to dissipate efficiently.

Avoid neglecting the importance of daily burping routines. New growers sometimes get impatient or forget, assuming that once buds are jarred, they can simply be left alone. Unfortunately, consistent burping is essential for preventing moisture buildup and giving off ammonia or other unwanted odors during curing. Early in the cure, more frequent burping—sometimes twice or thrice daily—can be necessary depending on moisture levels. Gradually, as buds stabilize and approach ideal moisture, burp intervals can be reduced to every few days. Pay attention to subtle changes in feel and smell within your jars to guide your burping schedule.

Finally, improper handling of buds after harvest and during curing can cause physical damage that affects quality. Crushing buds when packing jars tightly or frequently shaking containers to "mix" buds can break delicate trichomes that contain precious cannabinoids and terpenes. Loss of trichomes means less potent and less flavorful cannabis. Use gentle hands during trimming, transfer, and curing steps. If you notice a dusty residue left in jars or on your gloves, that's often trichomes breaking off. Respecting the physical integrity of your buds preserves their sensory qualities better through the curing process.

In summary, curing cannabis is a delicate dance that requires attention to moisture levels, temperature stability, airflow, and timing. Mold, over-drying, uneven curing, grassy flavors, and handling mistakes are the most common pitfalls, but they can all be managed with proper monitoring and adjustments. Stay patient and responsive during this final phase, and your efforts will be rewarded with smooth, flavorful buds that showcase the full character of your grow. Troubleshooting isn't just about fixing problems but also learning the subtle art of managing your unique harvest for maximum quality.

Chapter 24
Legal Considerations for Home Growing

Before you start planting seeds, it's crucial to understand the legal landscape surrounding home cultivation in your area. Laws vary widely—not just between states but sometimes between cities or counties—so knowing the local regulations on how many plants you can grow, where you're allowed to grow them, and any licensing or registration requirements is key to staying compliant and avoiding fines or legal trouble. Even if cannabis is legal where you live, there are often restrictions aimed at keeping your grow discreet and secure, protecting your personal privacy and safety. Being mindful of your neighbors and community standards can also help maintain good relations and prevent conflicts, which is just as important as following the letter of the law. Staying informed and up to date on legal changes lets you focus on cultivating quality buds without unnecessary stress, making your growing experience both rewarding and responsible.

Understanding Local Regulations and Limits

Before you even think about setting up your grow operation, it's crucial to get a solid grasp on the local rules that govern cannabis cultivation. These laws can vary widely—not just from one state to another, but also between cities and counties within the same state. What might be perfectly legal in one neighborhood could get you in serious trouble just a few miles down the road. So, starting your grow journey armed with knowledge about the specific restrictions where you live is an essential step.

Many places have strict limits not only on whether you can grow cannabis at home, but also how much you're allowed to cultivate. This typically covers the total number of plants, often distinguishing between mature and immature ones. Some local laws permit a handful of plants for personal use, while others might only allow seedlings or have no home growing allowed at all. It's important to note that these caps aren't always straightforward; they can change based on factors such as your residency status, whether you share your property with others, or if you live within certain municipal boundaries. Getting caught exceeding those limits can mean heavy fines, loss of your crop, or legal charges.

Another point to keep in mind is where you're allowed to grow your plants. Some ordinances mandate that cultivation must be done indoors, in secured and concealed environments, while others might have rules about outdoor grows—often requiring fences or other barriers to prevent public view and unauthorized access. Local laws can also include restrictions on how far your grow space must be from schools, parks, or places where children gather. These buffer zones are there to reduce exposure and prevent inadvertent access, so ignoring them is risky and often illegal.

One reason these laws might feel complex is that cannabis regulations change frequently. Lawmakers tweak rules to keep up with societal changes, public opinion, or new research findings. This means what's legal today might look very different in a year or two. This evolving landscape is why staying updated is just as important as understanding current laws. Local government websites, cannabis advocacy groups, and legal advisories are often good sources for the most recent information.

On top of quantity and location, some local governments regulate the type of cannabis you can grow. For example, certain jurisdictions might allow home cultivation but restrict plants to low-THC strains or those with knockdown medicinal uses only. Others might ban cultivation entirely from renters, allowing it only for homeowners. Restrictions like these prevent you from assuming that because growing is "legal" in your state, it's legal under any circumstance in your city or property type.

Besides knowing what's allowed, understanding the required security measures is equally important. You might have to lock your grow room or use surveillance cameras, especially if you live in a building with multiple residences. Many laws require your grow space to be inaccessible to the public and minors. While this may seem tedious, these rules are there to minimize theft, misuse, and any unwanted attention to your grow operation.

It's also essential to be aware of how local law enforcement typically enforces these rules. In some places, officers may be proactive in inspecting properties where unauthorized grows are suspected, while in others, enforcement might be more complaint-driven. Understanding enforcement practices can help you size up the risks and decide how strictly to invest in security and compliance. Being informed allows you to prepare your home grow in a way that's mindful of your community's expectations and legal landscape.

Sometimes the laws aren't just black and white—they leave gray areas that can trip up even experienced growers. For instance, the definition of a "mature" plant may vary in terms of when you need to count it toward your limit. Some regulations specify that a plant is mature only after it starts flowering, others consider size or age.

Misinterpreting these details can lead to inadvertent violations, so careful reading and, if needed, consulting with a local expert can save you headaches.

Another factor to consider is how these regulations tie into other parts of the legal system, like property rights and landlord-tenant agreements. Even if your local laws allow cultivation, your landlord might explicitly prohibit it in your lease. Failing to recognize this can lead to eviction or legal battles. Owners of multi-unit dwellings or homeowners associations may have rules against growing as well, so it pays to check those documents before investing time and resources into a grow setup.

For those who want to take their home growing a step further—perhaps preparing to sell or share their harvest, or even apply for a commercial license—there are separate layers of laws to master. While this section is focused on personal cultivation limits and regulations, it's wise to look ahead and see if local ordinances also address distribution, transport, or gifting of cannabis. Even for personal growers, understanding these boundaries can prevent unintended legal consequences.

Many enthusiasts underestimate the complexity of their local cannabis rules because they hear bits and pieces from friends or online forums, which often overlook smaller but critical details. There's no substitute for checking your city's municipal code or state's cannabis control board resources directly. If you're unsure or confused, seeking advice from cannabis-knowledgeable legal counsel can guide you in interpreting laws properly and keeping your growroom beyond reproach.

Scaling your cultivation operation without breaking the rules requires you to develop a habit of regularly reviewing local policies. Subscribe to newsletters, join neighborhood groups focused on cannabis advocacy, or participate in local discussions to stay in tune with shifts in regulation. Sometimes, public hearings or votes that change these laws occur without much fanfare, but they significantly impact what you can do legally. Proactivity will make the difference between a successful, long-term home grow and an abrupt shutdown that wipes out months of effort.

While rules can seem restrictive at first glance, they are often designed to balance your right to grow with the wider community's safety and order. Viewing these limits as guardrails rather than obstacles can help you approach your craft responsibly, with respect for neighbors and local authorities. By staying informed and compliant, you're better positioned not only to enjoy growing but also to advocate for positive change should the law need evolving in your area.

In short, understanding local regulations and limits isn't just about preventing legal trouble—it's about nurturing your home grow responsibly, sustainably, and smartly within the framework that's right for where you live. Doing the homework here lays the foundation for everything else you'll tackle in your cultivation journey, making the path to quality cannabis smoother and safer.

Licensing and Compliance Tips

When it comes to growing cannabis at home, understanding licensing and compliance is critical to keeping your operation legal and hassle-free. Even if your local laws permit personal cultivation, there are almost always rules and limits you need to follow. These can include the number of plants you're allowed to grow, where you can grow them, and sometimes even how you store your harvested product. Ignoring these regulations can lead to fines, confiscation of your crop, or worse. So, the best way to protect yourself and your investment is to stay informed and comply fully with local, state, and federal laws.

First things first: check if your state or city requires a cultivation license or permit, even for small home grows. While many places allow a certain number of plants without formal licensing, some jurisdictions require that growers register their grow, especially if you're cultivating more than the minimum personal-use limit. This registration often involves a simple application process, proof of residency, and an agreement to follow guidelines. Applying for a license or permit, when needed, shows authorities you're serious about operating responsibly—a factor that can save you headaches down the road.

Licenses, when required, also allow you access to legal protections and can be necessary if you want to expand your grow or eventually enter the commercial market. That said, don't assume a license means you're free to operate however you want. Compliance goes far beyond just holding a license. You will likely be responsible for regular inspections, keeping records, and abiding by rules related to signage, security, and odor control. Taking these compliance obligations seriously helps prevent complications and shows your commitment to being a trustworthy grower.

Security measures are one of the most common compliance points mentioned in licensing regulations. Many laws require that your grow space be limited in access—locked rooms or enclosed areas where unauthorized people, especially minors, can't get in. This is especially important if you live with family members or in shared housing. Beyond physical security, some areas want you to minimize external visibility of your plants to neighbors or passersby. This can include keeping plants indoors or shaded outdoors so they're not easily spotted. Ignoring these rules could make your grow a target for theft or complaints.

Another important compliance tip relates to the quantity and quality limits set by your jurisdiction. While home grows are often capped at a handful of plants, exceeding those limits can shift your operation from a personal grow into a commercial one, which comes with a completely different regulatory landscape. Some states also limit the weight or volume of usable cannabis you can possess from your home grow. Keep in mind that penalties for overproduction vary but often include the loss of your plants and legal fines.

Staying organized and documenting essential grow information can make licensing and compliance much easier. Keeping a detailed grow journal or log helps prove that your cultivation stays within legal boundaries. Record the number of plants, the stages of growth, and harvest amounts. If your local laws require it, keep receipts for seeds or clones purchased legally. This documentation can be invaluable if you ever have to show compliance to an inspector or law enforcement officer. It also helps you learn from each grow and improve your process.

Compliance goes beyond local rules, too. Remember that cannabis remains illegal under federal law in the United States, despite state-level legalization. While federal enforcement generally avoids home growers abiding by state laws, it's still wise to understand that federally enforced restrictions exist. Avoid transporting cannabis across state lines, and don't publicly advertise or distribute your home-grown product unless you're licensed to do so. Staying low-key and responsible can protect you from unexpected legal trouble.

Odor control is another practical tip related to compliance that can't be overlooked. Cannabis plants emit strong smells, especially during the flowering stage, which can cause issues with neighbors and lead to complaints that trigger law enforcement visits. Many local laws indirectly enforce odor control by requiring growers to take "reasonable measures" to avoid public nuisance. Using carbon filters, proper ventilation, and even installing smell-proof containers can keep your grow discreet and neighbor-friendly. Respecting your community helps create goodwill and lowers the risk of complaints.

For those considering expanding beyond personal cultivation, compliance typically becomes much more complex. Larger grows often require business licenses, tax registrations, zoning approvals, and compliance with health and safety codes. This section focuses mainly on home growing, but being aware of how these requirements differ can save you surprises if you decide to scale. Staying up-to-date on legislative changes is a must, too, since cannabis laws continue to evolve rapidly across jurisdictions.

One often overlooked compliance tip is to understand rules about sharing or gifting your home-grown cannabis. Some states allow gifting a limited amount to others, but selling without a license is almost always illegal. Make sure you know what your specific state permits to avoid accidental violations. Growing solely for personal use and refraining from unlicensed distribution are the safest bets when it comes to staying within legal limits.

Additionally, staying informed about environmental compliance matters can protect you as well. Some regions now regulate water usage, waste disposal, and energy consumption related to cannabis cultivation. Maintaining eco-friendly practices like water recycling, avoiding chemical runoff, and using energy-efficient equipment benefits both the environment and your standing with local authorities. Sustainable growing isn't only good for the planet—it can keep you compliant with emerging regulations targeting resource management.

Finally, take advantage of resources offered by local governments or cannabis advocacy groups. Many states provide online portals with up-to-date laws, application forms, and FAQs for growers. Industry forums, newsletters, and informational seminars often cover licensing procedures and compliance obligations in detail. Reaching out to these sources can save time and reduce the frustration of navigating complex rules on your own. Compliance doesn't have to feel intimidating if you stay proactive and informed.

In summary, the best licensing and compliance strategy for home growers is to know your local laws well, keep thorough records, maintain security and discretion, and always operate within the legal limits set by your jurisdiction. Following these guidelines not only protects you legally but also supports responsible and respectable cultivation within your community. Growing cannabis at home should be a positive and rewarding experience—

adhering to licensing and compliance standards helps ensure it stays that way for years to come.

Staying Safe and Respectful in Your Community

Growing cannabis at home comes with a unique blend of excitement and responsibility. Beyond the practical aspects of cultivation, it's just as important to stay mindful of your surroundings and how your activities might impact those around you. Being a cannabis grower doesn't mean operating in isolation—your neighbors, local community, and neighborhood atmosphere all play a role in creating a safe, respectful environment. This means taking proactive steps that foster trust, avoid conflicts, and keep your hobby within the bounds of respect for others.

First and foremost, one of the biggest concerns when growing cannabis at home is odor control. The distinctive smell of flowering cannabis can travel surprisingly far, and not everyone in your community may appreciate it. This is especially true in areas where cannabis cultivation is still a sensitive topic. To prevent any unwanted attention or complaints, investing in proper ventilation and air filtration systems—such as activated carbon filters—can drastically reduce odor. Managing smell not only protects your privacy but also shows consideration for neighbors who might not share your enthusiasm.

Another key aspect of staying respectful involves keeping your garden discreet and secure. Visibility matters a lot; you want to avoid creating a spectacle that might make neighbors feel uncomfortable or suspicious. For outdoor growers, using natural barriers like fences, trees, or shrubbery can help shield plants from view. Indoors, ensuring your grow lights aren't visible from windows and that any equipment noise is minimized will go a long way toward reducing disturbances. Keeping your grow discreet also has an added benefit: it reduces the risk of theft or vandalism, helping maintain your cultivation's safety.

Community relationships can make or break your home-growing experience. When possible, establish open and honest communication with your neighbors. Sometimes a simple conversation explaining that you're growing legally, for personal use, and taking measures to minimize any inconvenience can help clear the air and build goodwill. No one likes surprises, especially when it comes to cannabis. Demonstrating that you're responsible and respectful can prevent misunderstandings before they start. If a neighbor raises concerns, listening carefully and responding thoughtfully is essential. Showing empathy fosters trust, even if opinions differ.

Legal compliance forms the foundation of staying safe. Adhering strictly to your state or local regulations is not only about avoiding penalties but also about showing that you're a respectful member of your community. Overstepping limits—like growing more plants than allowed or failing to keep your cultivation secure—can quickly alienate neighbors and attract unwanted attention from law enforcement. Being aware of your jurisdiction's rules on plant counts, licensing, and permissible growing locations helps maintain your legitimacy and protects you from potential conflicts.

Don't underestimate the role of environmental responsibility either. Waste from growing operations, such as discarded plant material or excess nutrients, can create nuisances if not handled properly. Composting organic waste or disposing of it according to local guidelines demonstrates respect for community cleanliness and environmental health. Similarly, conserving water and managing odors also shows you care about minimizing your ecological footprint. Responsible cultivation blends seamlessly with being a responsible neighbor.

Security goes beyond just hiding your plants. Keeping your grow area locked and inaccessible to unauthorized people, especially children and pets, helps prevent accidents and unwanted exposure. Posting discreet signage to indicate the presence of a secured area is often recommended and can deter potential trespassers. If you live in shared housing or a multi-unit building, this takes on added importance, as careless access could jeopardize your entire community's peace of mind.

At the heart of respect is acknowledging that growing cannabis, though legal in many places, remains a personal choice that might not align with everyone's beliefs or comfort levels. Maintaining an attitude of humility and discretion protects your relationships and your ability to continue growing without friction. Remember, respect isn't just about avoiding problems—it's about fostering a positive atmosphere where your passion for growing can thrive alongside your community's well-being.

Cultivating cannabis can bring people together, too. If you're comfortable and it's appropriate in your community, sharing knowledge or even a small portion of your harvest can build camaraderie. Participating in local discussions or cannabis groups helps normalize the activity and educates others about responsible practices. When growers become active, respectful members of their community, they help dismantle stigma and create a more supportive environment for everyone.

In sum, staying safe and respectful means thinking beyond just your plants. It means managing odor, maintaining discretion, following laws, securing your garden, and nurturing good neighborly relations. These efforts aren't just about avoiding trouble—they're about building a sustainable lifestyle where home growing is as much about being a responsible member of your community as it is about cultivating your own high-quality cannabis. Taking these principles to heart will make your growing journey smoother, safer, and far more rewarding.

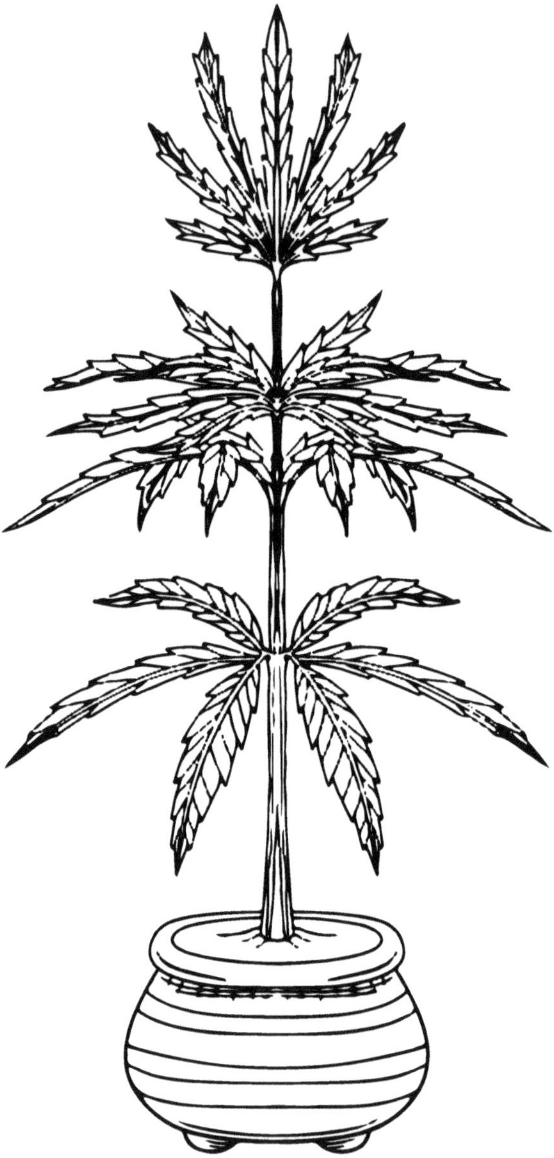

Chapter 25
Troubleshooting and Problem Prevention

Every grower hits a snag now and then, but the key to success lies in spotting issues early and preventing them before they become serious. Developing a routine for monitoring your plants—checking leaves, stems, and soil—helps catch problems like nutrient imbalances or pest infestations right away. Keeping a detailed grow journal can transform your approach by tracking what works and what doesn't, giving you valuable insights for future cycles. Learning from mistakes, adjusting your environmental controls, and staying curious about new techniques are all part of building confidence and consistency. Remember, the goal is to create a proactive mindset that minimizes surprises and maximizes your plants' health and yield over time.

Preventing Common Growing Mistakes

Even with the best intentions and careful planning, cannabis cultivation can be riddled with pitfalls that jeopardize your crop's success. Preventing common growing mistakes is not just about avoiding loss—it's about setting yourself up for consistent, rewarding results season after season. Whether you're planting your first seed or looking to fine-tune your setup, identifying these errors early on can save time, money, and frustration. The key lies in understanding the recurring challenges that growers face and taking proactive steps to steer clear of them.

One of the most frequent missteps is rushing the process. Cultivation demands patience and attention to detail, from germination to harvest. Beginners, in particular, often want to speed things along—watering too frequently, overfeeding nutrients, or forcing flowering stages prematurely. Plants don't respond well to these hurried interventions. Instead of pushing growth, rushing can cause stress, nutrient lockouts, or root problems that stunt development. It's better to allow the plant to progress naturally, keeping an eye on its signals while sticking to tried and true schedules for watering, feeding, and lighting.

Another major source of difficulty comes from over-complicating the environment. While it might be tempting to tweak every variable at once—humidity, temperature, pH, light intensity—this approach often backfires. Cannabis is resilient but thrives best in stable conditions. Dramatic daily swings or constant fiddling with settings can confuse plants and make diagnosing issues harder. Beginners especially benefit from starting simple: keep temperature consistent, maintain moderate humidity, and monitor pH closely but don't obsess over perfect numbers. Once you gain experience, slow adjustments become easier to manage.

Not understanding your water quality is a surprisingly common blunder. Tap water might contain chlorine, chloramine, or excessive minerals that affect soil chemistry and root health. Neglecting this can lead to nutrient lockout or toxic buildup in the growing medium. Many growers overlook testing their water or treating it before use. Investing in a basic water testing kit can reveal issues that inhibit growth, allowing you to adjust with filters, dechlorination methods, or water additives to create an ideal watering solution.

One of the trickiest mistakes involves improper nutrient management. Both underfeeding and overfeeding can cause significant setbacks. Cannabis plants have specific nutrient needs that fluctuate throughout the vegetative and flowering stages, and they respond poorly to extremes. Overfeeding can cause nutrient burn, presenting as yellowing or browning leaf tips that weaken the plant. On the flip side, underfeeding results in nutrient deficiencies that slow growth and reduce bud size. Regularly monitoring the plants and adjusting feeding schedules based on clear signs is pivotal.

Failing to calibrate light distance and intensity can also impair development. Lights that are too close can burn fans, while lights placed too far reduce photosynthesis efficiency. Different grow lights—whether LEDs, HPS, or CFLs—have unique heat outputs and penetration levels. Matching the light setup to your grow space and plant stages helps prevent stress and maximizes energy use. For example, young seedlings and clones need gentler, lower intensity light, while mature plants benefit from stronger illumination at the right distance.

One particularly sneaky area of error is neglecting the importance of airflow. Stagnant air around plants increases the risk of mold, mildew, and pest infestations. Ironically, many beginners focus on light and water but forget that proper ventilation is equally vital for a healthy environment. Good airflow helps maintain consistent temperature and humidity while strengthening plant stems. Whether growing indoors or outdoors, ensure your setup allows for adequate circulation. Using fans and exhaust systems prevents hotspots and keeps oxygen flowing where roots and leaves can thrive.

Another common trouble spot is soil choice and pot selection. Using poor quality or inappropriate soil can lead to drainage problems, root rot, and nutrient imbalances. Heavy, compacted soils don't let roots breathe enough and trap excess moisture, inviting fungal issues. On the other hand, overly light or sandy mixes won't retain enough water or nutrients. The right balance is crucial: soils that hold moisture but drain well, enriched with organic matter for sustained feeding. Similarly, pots that are too small stunt root growth, while those too large may lead to overwatering mistakes.

Ignoring the importance of cleanliness and hygiene is a silent culprit in many grow rooms. Pathogens and pests often hitch a ride in dust, on hands, or through contaminated tools. Failure to clean equipment regularly and sterilize equipment between grows can lead to persistent infestations that reduce yield or even ruin entire batches. Maintaining a clean grow space, washing hands before handling plants, and sanitizing scissors and pots are simple practices that pay huge dividends.

Misjudging the timing of key stages such as feeding adjustments, pruning, or switching light cycles can also backfire. Young plants, for example, don't benefit from high nitrates designed for heavy vegetative growth, while pushing flowering too fast stresses plants and lowers bud quality. Pruning at the wrong time can shock a plant or leave it vulnerable to pathogens. Learning to read your plants—watching for clear signs of readiness rather than guessing—helps avoid these timing pitfalls.

Lastly, one frequently underestimated mistake is insufficient record-keeping. Skipping detailed notes on everything from feeding schedules, light cycles, environmental conditions, and plant reactions leaves you flying blind when issues arise. Without data, it becomes guesswork to diagnose problems or improve success in future grows. A simple grow journal or log, updated regularly, is an invaluable tool to track what works and what doesn't. Many growers find it reveals patterns and helps them fine-tune their personal approach over time.

In summary, preventing common growing mistakes centers on respect for the plant's rhythms, consistent environment, and thorough observation. Avoid rushing, maintain stable conditions, and learn the intricacies of your setup before experimenting wildly. Focus on proper watering and feeding, provide the right light and airflow, and don't overlook sanitation and record-keeping. These steps create a solid foundation that empowers both new and intermediate growers to produce healthier plants and better yields. In the world of cannabis cultivation, prevention truly beats cure, making every grow run smoother and more enjoyable.

Creating a Grow Journal and Tracking Progress

One of the most valuable yet often overlooked tools for any cannabis grower is a grow journal. Whether you're just starting out or have been cultivating for years, keeping a detailed record of your grow sessions can dramatically improve your results. Think of your grow journal as a personalized guidebook that evolves with your experience, helping you spot patterns, troubleshoot problems, and optimize your techniques over time.

When you first set up your grow journal, consider what information will be most useful to track. Start with basic details like strain names, seed sources, and germination dates. From there, note environmental conditions such as light schedules, temperature, humidity, and ventilation adjustments. Tracking watering and feeding schedules can reveal a lot when it comes to diagnosing deficiencies or overfeeding. These notes become invaluable in understanding how your plants respond to specific conditions and changes.

The importance of consistency can't be overstated. Logging your observations daily—or at least every time you interact with your plants—creates a clear timeline. This ongoing record lets you pinpoint exactly when a change occurred, whether it was the introduction of a new nutrient, a shift in lighting, or the appearance of early signs of pests or stress. Instead of guessing what caused a problem, you have hard evidence to support your decisions.

Besides environmental factors, your grow journal should include detailed observations of plant health and behavior. Describe leaf color and texture, the presence of any spots or deformities, and overall plant vigor. During the flowering stage, track bud development, noting size, density, and any issues like mold or nutrient burn. The more specific and descriptive you are, the easier it becomes to compare grows and hone in on what's working best.

Photos are another excellent addition. Modern smartphones make it simple to snap quick shots of your plants throughout each growth phase. Date-stamped photos provide a visual timeline that's often more revealing than written notes alone. You might notice subtle differences in leaf growth or color that you didn't catch in person but become clear when reviewing images side by side. Just be sure to organize and label photos clearly so you can quickly find them when needed.

Tracking progress isn't only about problem-solving—it's also a powerful motivator. When you flip back through previous logs and see how much your skills and plants have improved, it fuels enthusiasm to keep pushing forward. Especially when a particular method or nutrient regimen yields bigger, denser buds, having detailed proof of that success encourages you to replicate and build on what you've learned.

Setting goals is a natural extension of maintaining a grow journal. If you aim to improve potency, increase yield, or reduce pest issues, document baseline data and measure progress against those targets. For example, note your harvest weights, average THC testing results if available, or frequency of pest outbreaks. Over time, you'll build a rich database of grow cycles that clearly map your journey toward better cannabis cultivation.

Digital or analog formats both have their merits. Some growers prefer physical notebooks for the tactile satisfaction and ease of jotting things down without distractions. Others opt for digital solutions—spreadsheets, grow journal apps, or simple note-taking software—which offer search functions, cloud backups, and easy photo integration. Find whichever format you're more comfortable with and that you'll consistently use. The key is maintaining regular entries.

Don't underestimate the value of detailed notes even for what might seem like minor tweaks. Changing your light height by just a few inches or experimenting with a new pruning technique can be game-changers when carefully documented. Over multiple grows, you'll develop your own playbook customized for your unique setup—weather, space constraints, and plant genetics all influence what works best.

One of the benefits of a grow journal is its role in preventing recurring problems. If you learn to catch early signs of deficiencies, pests, or stress symptoms, recording these instances helps you identify the conditions that caused them. This insight lets you avoid making the same mistakes, saving time, money, and plants. Rather than repeating trial and error blindly, you gain a strategic edge by learning from your own history.

Additionally, a grow journal can become a resource to share with other cultivators or mentors. When you're able to clearly explain what you've tried, what went right, and what didn't, it facilitates better advice and support. Whether participating in online forums, grower clubs, or discussions with professionals, having detailed records elevates your credibility and helps pinpoint solutions faster.

Another aspect worth mentioning is how journals serve as a safety net when life interferes with your growing routine. Unexpected absences or busy periods can lead to missed watering or feedings, which are easier to manage when you have precise records of what was done and when. This way, you can quickly assess whether your plants need catch-up care or if conditions remain stable enough to withstand temporary neglect.

Many growers eventually expand their journals beyond basic observations to include experimental data. You might test how different nutrient combinations affect growth or how specific pruning techniques impact yields. Recording variables and results systematically turns your grow journal into a mini research lab, advancing your knowledge and skill set organically.

Remember, the primary goal of creating and maintaining a grow journal is to improve your grow's consistency and quality. It encourages a mindset of curiosity, diligence, and accountability. Over time, your journal becomes a tailored blueprint that guides decision-making in every phase—vegetative, flowering, harvest, and curing—helping avoid the pitfalls that catch many new growers off guard.

In summary, the practice of journaling transforms cannabis cultivation from a guessing game into a scientific and artistic pursuit. By carefully tracking progress and challenges, you're empowered to adapt and optimize your grow environment and techniques. This informed approach increases the odds of healthy plants, bigger yields, and a more satisfying harvest.

Resources for Continued Learning and Support

Growing cannabis can be both incredibly rewarding and occasionally challenging. Even after working through the steps, questions pop up and obstacles appear. That's why tapping into reliable resources designed for ongoing learning is so important in your cultivation journey. Whether you're a total newbie or someone who's grown several harvests, having a solid support system and accessible knowledge at your fingertips helps prevent frustration and accelerates improvement.

First, leaning on knowledgeable communities—both online and offline—offers a tremendous advantage. Forums and social media groups dedicated to cannabis growing provide lively spaces where enthusiasts share real-world experiences and troubleshoot common problems together. Platforms like Reddit's r/microgrowery, GrowDiaries, and specific Facebook groups host thousands of growers exchanging tips on everything from seed selection to pest control. These conversations can expose you to diverse perspectives and solutions you might not find in standard guides.

Besides active discussion groups, a trove of high-quality, continuously updated educational content exists in the form of articles, videos, and podcasts. Many successful growers and industry experts share video tutorials covering advanced techniques such as plant training, nutrient adjustments, or lighting hacks. Channels on YouTube like "From Seed to Stoned" or "Mr. Canucks Grow" break complex topics into manageable lessons, which makes learning on your own schedule a breeze. Similarly, podcasts focused on cannabis cultivation dive into emerging trends, regulatory updates, and sustainability practices that keep you informed and motivated.

Books and eBooks still hold tremendous value in this niche. Numerous authors, often with years of hands-on growing experience, have penned comprehensive guides that go beyond basics and delve into nuanced challenges beginners often face. These resources are carefully structured to build your foundational knowledge and offer step-by-step approaches to diagnosing problems. Whether you prefer printed editions for easy reference or digital versions accessible on the go, having expert-curated information structured systematically helps enormously when trying to troubleshoot stubborn issues.

Beyond just books and online groups, many growers find workshops and local meetups incredibly beneficial. Cannabis cultivation classes or seminars can provide hands-on experience and allow you to connect directly with experts. These gatherings sometimes happen in community centers, specialty garden shops, or even at larger cannabis expositions. Participating adds a valuable layer of education since you can ask questions face-to-face and see techniques demonstrated live. Plus, the social aspect encourages sharing knowledge and building friendships within the enthusiast network.

A dynamic grow journal is another underutilized but powerful resource. Keeping detailed records of your plants' progress, environmental conditions, feeding schedules, and any problems you notice creates a personalized database of what works and what doesn't in your unique environment. Over time, this record becomes an invaluable tool to catch patterns, anticipate difficulties, and fine-tune your approach. Many growers supplement traditional notebooks with digital apps designed specifically for cannabis cultivation tracking, offering reminders and data visualization tools.

When you run into unexpected issues—like mysterious leaf discoloration or sudden pest outbreaks—consulting diagnostic charts and troubleshooting guides can quickly point you in the right direction. Many reputable websites and grow manuals feature comprehensive symptom checklists paired with recommended corrective actions. These resources are essential for identifying problems early, so you don't lose big chunks of your crop to preventable mistakes. Bookmarking these practical guides ensures fast solutions rather than spending hours guessing or waiting for harmful issues to worsen.

Access to professional grow consultations is becoming more common, especially as cannabis cultivation steadily gains mainstream acceptance. Some companies and experienced cultivators offer personalized services, from virtual coaching sessions to in-person facility visits. These experts can analyze your setup and plant health, then tailor advice to your specific challenges—something that generic advice can't always provide. Though this option might involve a cost, it's often worth the investment when tackling complex problems, especially if maximizing quality and yield is your goal.

Maintaining strong ties with quality suppliers also supports continued success. Trusted vendors not only provide top-notch seeds, nutrients, and equipment but often supply how-to guides, troubleshooting articles, and customer service assistance. Building relationships with these suppliers can lead to insider tips or early access to innovative products that enhance your grow operation. Relying on reputable sources reduces the risk of encountering subpar materials that might cause cultivation setbacks.

Legal resources play a critical role too. Cannabis laws change frequently and can vary widely by jurisdiction. Staying updated through government websites, industry newsletters, or legal advisory services prevents unintentional violations that could jeopardize your growing privileges. Some nonprofit organizations also offer free or low-cost legal guidance tailored specifically for home growers, making this an invaluable safety net for responsible cultivation.

Lastly, don't underestimate the power of curiosity and experimentation fueled by continuous education. The cannabis growing landscape evolves rapidly with new strains, tools, and techniques emerging regularly. Subscribing to newsletters from cultivator networks, industry experts, or seed banks ensures you're among the first to hear about breakthroughs. This proactive learning mindset cultivates resilience, enabling you to adapt and thrive through challenges rather than being slowed down by them.

In summary, tapping into a rich ecosystem of resources—community networks, multimedia content, books, workshops, journals, diagnostic tools, professional advice, trusted suppliers, and legal information—builds a strong foundation to support your growth as a cultivator. These ongoing learning supports empower you to face problems head-on, prevent future issues, and refine your skills continuously. Cannabis cultivation is both an art and a science, and with the right resources, you can approach each phase with confidence and enthusiasm to cultivate top-tier crops from seed to harvest.

Conclusion

Growing cannabis at home is more than just a hobby—it's an evolving craft, one that combines science, patience, and a deep appreciation for the plant itself. Throughout this book, the journey from seed to harvest was laid out carefully to guide both newcomers and seasoned cultivators alike. If you've followed along, you now possess a toolkit filled with knowledge on the essentials: how to select the right seeds, manage environmental factors, nurture plant health, and handle post-harvest processes. But beyond just technique, growing cannabis is about developing an intuitive understanding of your plants and adapting to their needs as they grow. That's where true mastery begins.

One of the biggest takeaways is the importance of patience. Cannabis cultivation can't be rushed without risking quality or yield. Each stage of growth demands attention and care, often with subtle adjustments that only come with experience and observation. Whether dealing with lighting, nutrients, or pest management, no single tactic guarantees success on its own. It's the combination of consistent effort, learning from mistakes, and tuning your approach to your unique environment that makes all the difference. This book aimed to remove the guesswork and give a clear path forward, but the grower's touch is what ultimately transforms a garden into a thriving, potent crop.

There's also something empowering about growing cannabis within the limits of the law, responsibly and sustainably. Being mindful of your local regulations not only keeps you out of trouble but encourages better stewardship of the resources and spaces you work with. Sustainable growing practices, as explored earlier, are about more than reducing waste—they're about ensuring you can continue to cultivate successfully for years to come without compromising the environment. The balance between maximizing yields and respecting natural cycles fosters a deeper respect for the entire growing process.

Technology and equipment have come a long way in assisting home growers, but this book emphasized that tools alone don't create quality harvests. Understanding the plant's biology, its needs during each phase, and how environmental variables influence growth creates a solid foundation that technology can then enhance. Whether you're setting up a modest indoor grow tent or cultivating in a backyard garden, the core principles remain the same. Tailoring equipment choices to your individual style and budget makes cannabis cultivation both accessible and scalable.

The varied topics covered—from choosing the right strain for your goals to mastering watering schedules—underscore the complexity and nuance of cannabis growing. But complexity shouldn't be intimidating. Instead, think of it as a series of manageable steps. When broken down, each challenge becomes an opportunity to learn more and get better results. For beginners especially, starting with simple setups and gradually introducing advanced techniques will build confidence and prevent overwhelm. For intermediate growers, refining and experimenting with advanced lighting, training methods, or organic nutrient setups is where real breakthroughs happen.

Another critical insight is the value of observation. Cannabis plants communicate their needs through changes in color, leaf texture, and growth patterns. Becoming fluent in this language lets you catch nutrient deficiencies, pest invasions, or environmental stress early—before they cause significant damage. Early intervention is often what separates a mediocre harvest from an exceptional one. This book aimed to provide the knowledge and checklists to spot these warning signs and act promptly. It's about turning problems into learning moments instead of catastrophic failures.

Harvest time marks both a culmination and a new beginning. Knowing when to cut your buds and how to cure them properly can amplify potency, flavor, and smoothness of the final product. These post-harvest steps are often underestimated but critically shape the quality you get to enjoy. Patient drying and curing, along with proper storage, help lock in the fruits of your labor for months or even years. Mastering these phases ensures that the effort you pour into cultivation translates into a superior experience when consuming or sharing your harvest.

Growing cannabis isn't just about the end product; it's about embracing the entire journey—from planting that tiny seed to enjoying the fruits of your patience. Each cycle teaches valuable lessons about biology, timing, and perseverance. The sense of accomplishment that comes with harvesting your own cannabis can't be overstated. It's a unique blend of pride, satisfaction, and connection to the plant and your environment.

As the cannabis landscape continues to evolve with new strains, technologies, and legal frameworks, staying informed and adaptable will serve you well. This book serves as both a foundation and a springboard, encouraging ongoing learning and experimentation. Growing is part science, part art, and part personal expression. Your garden responds to your environment, choices, and care in ways that create a distinct signature unique to your hands and space.

Ultimately, success in cannabis cultivation is a blend of dedication, knowledge, creativity, and respect for the plant's cycles. Whether your goal is to produce high-quality flowers for personal use or develop skills for potential future ventures, fostering a mindful and informed approach will elevate your results. The path covered here lays out the stepping stones, but your passion and persistence will shape your outcome. Keep learning, observing, and innovating with each grow—because that's where the true reward lies.

So, take this blueprint and make it your own. Grow with intention, appreciate the nuances of the plant, and don't shy away from challenges—they are part of the process that leads to becoming a confident, skilled cannabis cultivator. The knowledge you've gained empowers you to grow legally, safely, and successfully, and that's the foundation for enjoying cannabis cultivation as an enriching and fulfilling practice for years to come.

Appendix

This appendix serves as a handy resource hub to support your journey as a cannabis grower, whether you're just starting out or looking to finesse your cultivation skills. Inside, you'll find practical tools like sample grow logs and checklists that help keep your grow organized and efficient, along with a glossary clarifying essential cannabis growing terms to bridge any knowledge gaps that might pop up. Additionally, we've compiled a list of recommended resources and trusted suppliers to connect you with quality gear and seeds, so you can confidently source what you need without guesswork. Think of this section as your quick-reference guide to complement everything covered in the main chapters, giving you extra confidence and support as you strive to produce top-shelf cannabis right at home.

Glossary of Cannabis Growing Terms

Getting familiar with the language of cannabis cultivation will make your growing journey smoother and more enjoyable. This glossary covers key terms every grower—whether just starting out or already experienced—should know to successfully raise healthy, potent cannabis plants. Understanding these words helps you follow instructions, troubleshoot issues, and communicate confidently within the cannabis community.

- **Autoflower**: A type of cannabis plant that automatically begins flowering after a certain age, regardless of light cycles. Great for beginners and quick harvests.
- **Clone**: A cutting taken from a healthy "mother" plant that will grow into a genetically identical cannabis plant. Cloning speeds up growing and preserves preferred traits.
- **Flush**: The process of watering plants with pure water (no nutrients) for a period before harvest. This helps remove excess salts and improves flavor and smoothness.
- **Feminized Seeds**: Seeds bred to produce only female plants, which are the ones that develop

buds rich in cannabinoids. Saves time and effort compared to growing regular seeds.

- **Glasshouse**: A greenhouse-style structure used for growing cannabis, offering natural light while protecting plants from outdoor elements.
- **Hydroponics**: A soilless growing method where plants grow in nutrient-rich water solutions. It can speed growth and increase yields but requires careful monitoring.
- **Indica**: A cannabis variety known for its relaxing and sedative effects. Indicas tend to have broader leaves and shorter, bushier growth patterns.
- **Light Cycle**: The schedule of light and darkness a plant receives, typically 18+ hours of light during vegetative stage and 12 hours during flowering indoors.
- **Nutrients**: Essential minerals and elements like nitrogen, phosphorus, and potassium that cannabis needs to grow strong and produce buds.
- **Pistils**: The hair-like structures on flowering female cannabis plants that catch pollen. Their color changes (white to orange/brown) help indicate plant maturity.
- **PH**: A measure of how acidic or alkaline your water or soil is. Cannabis plants prefer slightly acidic conditions, usually between 6.0 and 7.0.

- **Photoperiod**: A type of cannabis that flowers based on changes in light cycle length, unlike autoflowers which flower by age.
- **Pruning**: Trimming away leaves and branches to improve airflow, light penetration, and redirect the plant's energy for better yields.
- **Resin**: Sticky glandular secretion on cannabis buds containing cannabinoids and terpenes—the compounds responsible for potency, aroma, and effects.
- **Sexing**: Identifying male and female cannabis plants before flowering to prevent unwanted pollination and seed production.
- **Sativa**: A cannabis variety associated with uplifting and energetic effects. Sativas usually have thinner leaves and taller, lankier growth habits.
- **Stoma (plural: stomata)**: Tiny pores on leaves that allow gas exchange—letting plants breathe, sweat, and stay cool.
- **Trichomes**: Tiny, crystal-like structures on buds and leaves packed with cannabinoids and terpenes. Their color and clarity indicate harvest readiness.
- **Vegetative Stage**: The growth phase when the plant focuses on developing stems and leaves before flowering starts.

- **Yield**: The final amount of cannabis buds harvested, often measured by weight. Growers aim to maximize yield without sacrificing quality.

Keep this glossary handy as you grow to quickly reference terms and keep your cultivation knowledge sharp. Mastering these basics sets the foundation for success and helps you make the most of every step in your growing adventure.

Recommended Resources and Suppliers

Navigating the world of cannabis cultivation can be overwhelming, especially when it comes to finding trustworthy resources and reliable suppliers. Whether you're just starting out or have been growing for years, having access to the right products and information can make all the difference in your success. While this book covers many practical growing techniques and essential knowledge, this section focuses on guiding you toward reputable resources where you can source quality materials and deepen your learning.

One of the most valuable assets in any grower's toolkit is good information. Numerous online communities and forums offer excellent advice, shared experiences, and support from fellow cultivators. Websites like GrowDiaries, Rollitup, and Reddit's r/ microgrowery provide a wealth of user-generated content and discussions that can help answer specific questions or troubleshoot issues when they arise. These platforms are great for real-time feedback and learning from a diverse range of growers, from hobbyists to seasoned professionals.

For more structured knowledge, well-regarded blogs and educational sites run by experienced growers and horticulturalists can be reliable sources. Some specialize in organic growing methods, while others focus on hydroponics or indoor cultivation. Following these can keep you up-to-date with new trends, advanced techniques, and equipment reviews. Staying plugged into these channels often offers early insights on innovations and best practices, which proves invaluable when tweaking your grow for better results.

When it comes to sourcing your supplies, choosing reputable vendors ensures you get high-quality products that perform as expected. For seeds, companies with transparent genetics and customer reviews stand out. Seed banks like ILoveGrowingMarijuana, Seedsman, and Herbies Seeds have earned solid reputations for shipping reliability and strain variety. Selecting feminized or autoflower seeds from respected suppliers reduces the risk of ending up with low-quality or misrepresented genetics—something every grower wants to avoid.

Besides seeds, quality soil, nutrients, and growing mediums form the backbone of a healthy cultivation environment. Brands such as FoxFarm, General Hydroponics, and Advanced Nutrients offer products specifically formulated for cannabis, tailored to its nuanced nutrient requirements throughout growth stages. Many growers find success pairing nutrient lines with their chosen soil or hydroponic setups. It's crucial to invest in proven products, even if they're slightly more expensive up front. Lower quality alternatives often result in nutrient imbalances or poor plant health, costing more time and money in the long run.

Lighting and environmental controls are another pillar of a great grow. Top-tier suppliers like Gavita, Mars Hydro, and Spider Farmer provide lighting solutions optimized for cannabis, balancing spectrum, intensity, and energy efficiency. Fans, carbon filters, and climate controllers are best obtained from specialized horticultural retailers rather than general hardware stores, as these offer gear designed to maintain ideal airflow and odor control within grow tents and rooms. Making sure these components are compatible and reliable will avoid frustrating setbacks, such as heat stress or pest infestations.

Beyond products, consider investing in good tools and accessories—pruners, magnifying lenses for trichome inspection, pH meters, and humidity controllers. Brands like Milwaukee Instruments and Bluelab produce accurate, durable meters favored by serious growers. While it might be tempting to cut costs here, precision tools are essential for monitoring and adjusting conditions that directly affect your harvest's quality and potency.

Many experienced cultivators also swear by growing journals and software to track their plants' progress. These resources support systematic data collection on feeding schedules, environmental changes, and growth milestones, which helps identify what worked and what didn't over multiple cycles. Some growers use apps like GrowBuddy or Leafly's Grow software to organize their notes and get strain-specific insights. Keeping detailed records is a habit that pays dividends by improving your efficiency and yield with each grow.

In addition to supplies and information, building a connection with local or online cannabis growing groups can be invaluable. These communities often arrange seed swaps, share cutting-edge techniques, and recommend trusted local suppliers you might not find on your own. And during times when laws and regulations shift, community support offers timely guidance on compliance and safety best practices—both crucial for responsible home cultivation.

For those seeking hands-on education beyond reading and forums, look for workshops and courses offered by cannabis horticulture schools or gardening centers in legal states. Some universities and private institutions now provide specialized cannabis cultivation training, covering everything from plant biology to commercial scale operations. Attending these can supercharge your skills and help you network with professional growers and industry experts.

Consider also subscribing to magazines or newsletters dedicated to cannabis culture and cultivation. Publications like High Times, Cannabis Business Times, and Growing for Market often include in-depth articles, product tests, and market trends that keep you informed about the broader cannabis landscape beyond your own grow room. This awareness can inspire innovation and motivate you to continuously evolve your skills and setup.

Lastly, one should always remain cautious with suppliers offering deals that seem too good to be true. It's wise to research vendors thoroughly—including reading customer reviews and looking for guarantees or return policies—before making significant investments. Remember that exceptional cannabis grows from consistent quality inputs paired with patience and attention, not from shortcuts or subpar components.

Choosing the right resources and suppliers lays the foundation for a successful cannabis cultivation journey. By leveraging trusted product brands, engaging with knowledgeable communities, and continuously educating yourself, you build a strong support system that elevates your growing experience. Whether you're sourcing a rare seed strain or upgrading your lighting system, knowing where to turn will keep your garden thriving and your passion fueled for harvest after harvest.

Sample Grow Logs and Checklists

Keeping detailed grow logs and using checklists can be game-changers when cultivating cannabis, no matter your experience level. Logging your grow activities allows you to track progress, identify patterns, and spot potential problems before they spiral out of control. Think of it as a personal journal dedicated solely to your plants' health and development, giving you a clear roadmap to replicate successes or tweak techniques for better results.

A solid grow log doesn't have to be complicated. Simple daily or weekly entries noting watering, feeding amounts, growth milestones, light cycles, and environmental conditions like temperature and humidity can make a huge difference. Consistency is key here. When you jot down what happened and how your plants responded, you build a valuable database of knowledge customized to your unique grow setup and strains.

For example, if you notice leaf discoloration or curling, having a recent log can help you connect those symptoms to recent changes, such as nutrient adjustments or environmental shifts. Over time, this data sharpens your intuition about when to intervene or change strategies, which leads to healthier plants and better yields.

Checklists complement grow logs by offering practical, straightforward steps to follow during each phase of growing. They work like a safety net ensuring critical tasks aren't forgotten in the hustle of daily maintenance. Prepping a checklist beforehand for stages like germination, vegetative growth, flowering, and harvesting can keep you organized and reduce stress.

For instance, a vegetative stage checklist might include verifying light schedules, checking soil moisture levels, inspecting plants for pests, and monitoring nutrient feedings. Crossing off these tasks daily instills a routine that establishes healthy habits and prevents overlooked details that could stunt plant development. Checklists also make training new growers easier, especially if you share growing responsibilities or want a consistent approach across multiple grows.

Besides the basics, customizing your logs and checklists according to your methods and goals enhances their usefulness. If you're experimenting with organic nutrients, you might want entries focused on soil amendments and their effects. If you grow indoors, logging light types and durations alongside ventilation adjustments can help fine-tune your environment.

Some growers prefer digital logs and checklists—using apps or spreadsheets that allow easy editing, filtering, and reminders. Others stick to old-school pen and paper, appreciating the tactile experience and simplicity. Whichever route you choose, the habit of logging and checking tasks regularly creates accountability and fosters ongoing improvement.

Another useful thing to include in your grow logs is daily observations on plant health and behavior. Are the leaves bright green or showing signs of nutrient deficiency? Is stretching occurring, indicating potential lighting issues? Are buds swelling as expected during flowering? These notes connect the dots between your care routine and the plant's response, helping avoid costly trial-and-error over multiple grow cycles.

Tracking environmental factors—temperature swings, humidity spikes, or airflow changes—is equally important. For instance, if your grow log shows a sudden rise in humidity and you later notice mold issues, you'll know exactly when and why it happened, allowing you to adjust setup or schedules moving forward. Detailed logs help you remain proactive rather than reactive.

Harvest checklists, in particular, help prepare you for one of the most crucial moments in cannabis cultivation. The right timing improves potency, flavor, and overall quality. Your checklist might include steps such as inspecting trichomes, trimming techniques, curing environment preparation, and storage solutions. Missing or rushing through any of these can diminish the hard work invested during previous growth stages.

It's also worthwhile to set weekly or biweekly review sessions for your logs and checklists. This isn't just about marking tasks done; it's your chance to analyze trends, refine your routines, and plan ahead. Are you noticing consistently under- or over-watering? Is your lighting schedule optimizing growth or causing stress? Did a particular nutrient formula yield better bud quality last cycle? These insights help evolve a more effective and personalized growing style.

In group grows or community gardens, grow logs and checklists become vital communication tools. Sharing entries helps coordinate efforts, spot problems earlier, and learn collectively from each cycle's successes and challenges. Collaboration raises the bar for everyone involved and deepens your connection to the growing community.

Finally, remember that patience and precision go hand-in-hand with successful cannabis cultivation. Your grow logs and checklists are your allies in this journey. They transform guesswork into data-driven decisions and chaotic routines into manageable, repeatable processes. By committing to these practices, you boost your chances of producing higher-quality cannabis with more confidence.

The key takeaway is that no grow is too small or too simple to document. Even a modest setup benefits from thoughtful tracking and planning. So start your grow log early, update it regularly, and tailor your checklists to suit your unique approach. The results will speak for themselves when you see healthier plants, bigger yields, and a smoother, more enjoyable growing experience.